PEAK PHYSIQUE

Published by Bloomsbury Publishing Plc
50 Bedford Square
London WC1B 3DP
www.bloomsbury.com

Bloomsbury is a trademark of Bloomsbury Publishing Plc

First edition 2015

ISBN (print): 978-1-4729-1257-2
ISBN (ePdf): 978-1-4729-1259-6
ISBN (EPUB): 978-1-4729-1258-9

A CIP catalogue record for this book is available from the British Library.

Acknowledgements
Produced by Lisa Purcell Editorial & Design
Photography by Jen Schmidt Photography
Commissioned by Kirsty Schaper
Models: Hollis Lance Liebman and Michelle Brooke

This book is produced using paper that is made from wood grown in managed, sustainable forests. It is
natural, renewable and recyclable. The logging and manufacturing processes conform to the environmental
regulations of the country of origin.

Typeset in Helvetica Neue and ITC Novarese by Lisa Purcell Editorial & Design, USA

Printed and bound in China by C&C Offset Printing Co.,LTD

10 9 8 7 6 5 4 3 2 1

PEAK PHYSIQUE

YOUR TOTAL BODY TRANSFORMATION

HOLLIS LANCE LIEBMAN

BLOOMSBURY

LONDON · NEW DELHI · NEW YORK · SYDNEY

CONTENTS

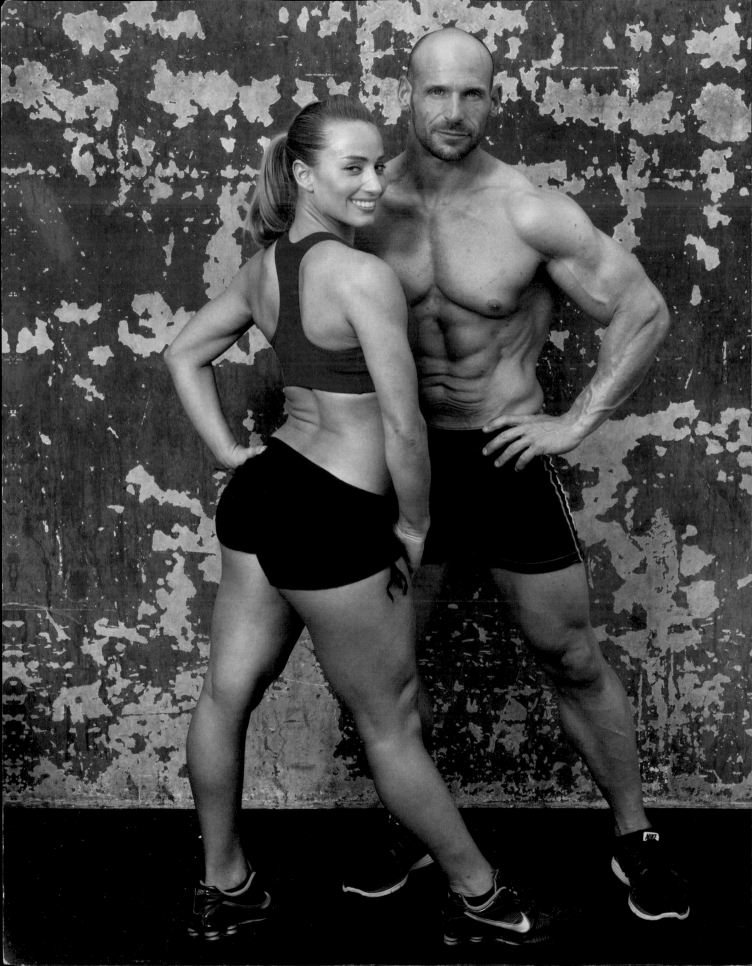

FOREWORD

I first met Hollis in the summer of 2005 when he approached me in an L.A. gym to tell me that he was a fan of my work. It didn't take me long to realize that he was a very interesting person and that I really liked him. Besides sharing the love of heavy metal music, tasteless jokes and the female form, we also shared the passion for helping people. Hollis truly cares and has made it his life's work and mission to help others better themselves, both mentally and physically.

Over the years, I have seen Hollis progress, and he is now nearing the top of his field. This book is not only the culmination of his many years in the fitness industry, but it's also the culmination of his studies on how to become one's best—starting with the mind.

I was surprised when I saw the layout for this book, not only because it rocks, but also because I'd never seen him in this kind of shape before. And it was because he executed with perfect precision his message, his plan. I asked what it took for him to get into that kind of shape, and he told me he had reset his mind and was reevaluating how he could become the best he could be.

Peak Physique stands on its own, is artistically ambitious and answers the decades-old questions of the what, the whom and the how to get there.

Trust this guy: he knows what he's doing, and he's the best in the world at what he does.

Chris Jericho
Tampa, Florida

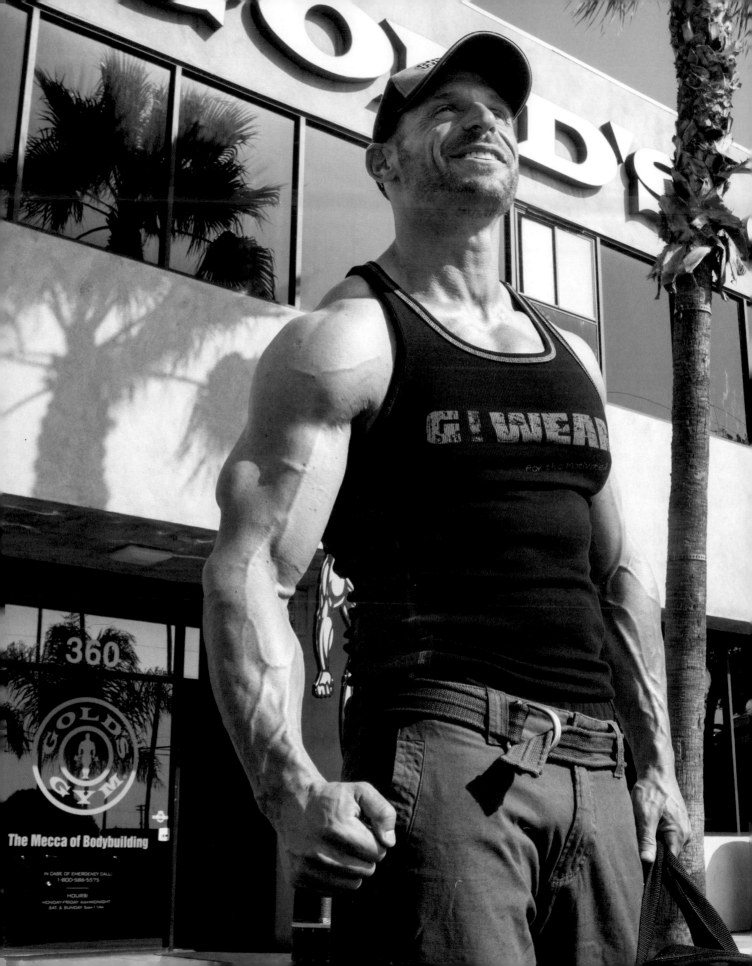

AN INVITE TO "RESETTING" YOU

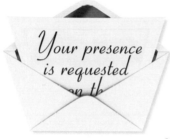

In the grand play list of reality, there exists more givens than just death and taxes. For in between, there's a never-ending list of items placed into the shopping cart that is life. Another errand to check off, another destination, another obstacle, and yes, another occasion or event that looms ahead, requiring your presence. A gathering, a visit, an organized bundling of activities and persons, places and things on a given day where your attendance is cordially requested. And amid most of our hyperbusy lives in this always-on, social media world we live in today, the thought of making an appearance at less than our best is most certainly less than appealing.

As children, if we'd woken up on a school day with an overwhelmingly large spot on our face or less-than-fabulous haircut for Monday-morning classes or, for some of us, after-school activities, then it was indeed too bad. No excuses—we still had to go. But as adults, we have choices, which include, quite simply, not attending.

THE DREADED INVITATION

Say you've been invited to a wedding, but your trousers don't quite zip up or the top button on your dress shirt won't close without a shoe horn, and a trip to the "big and tall" shop is too far out of the way? Or your class reunion is looming and your favorite cocktail dress is bursting at the seams, and you just threw out the latest plus-size catalog? Victoria's Secret seems to be just that—a place only skinny girls know the password to. No problem, you just tell yourself that you won't attend the event. Or maybe, for some, you will attend, as you no longer care how you look or feel and there is nothing to be done to change it.

But how we look on the outside often dictates how we feel inside, or at least offers more than a glimpse of what is really going on within us. In my own life, I am an author and a personal trainer. I make my living helping others achieve their physique goals. And yet, for nearly two years, I had—at best—a very difficult time getting into and maintaining proper shape. Did it affect my self-esteem? You bet. Do I blame others? No. Only myself. Yes, I was in a toxic relationship, and yes, eating was one of the few pleasures afforded to me at the time. And so I overcompensated with food in order to feel something, anything, daily. Did I skip events I was eagerly invited to? Unfortunately, yes. I was unhappy with both the inward and outward me, and often the only public exposure I would subject myself to was a fast-food drive-thru, where I'd put in my order with three small dogs fighting for the most advantageous position for snatching grease-laden, salty fries.

TIME TO RESET

So what changed between then and now, aside from dropping a lot of body fat? Perhaps the grandest event of them all: Life. I was newly single and desperately needed my self-esteem back. Like many, I wanted to feel comfortable leaving the light on when resuming the bed dance with a future partner. I believe there is a rock-bottom point, or a switch that must be hit in the human brain when imminent and impending change is in order, when we agree that our current self just doesn't represent who we really are and that we demand better of ourselves for ourselves.

And so the genesis of this book that you now hold in your hands began as a tale of revenge. Not revenge against my ex, but instead revenge against myself—the me who enabled and masterminded my fall from grace.

I realized that sometimes in a relationship we can get lazy. We stop with the care and maintenance that our significant other may have fallen for in the first place.

No one ever placed a gun to my head and forced me to overeat and put on the pounds. Although there was definitely something missing from that relationship in order for me to overcompensate with food, I alone did it to myself. And I alone would stage a return to and beyond my former glory.

And so, as the meals and training sessions turned into days and then weeks, I knew I had to not only document the journey, but also define and map it so that others could follow my path and free themselves too. Scheduling an actual photo shoot in which I would appear beyond my normal roles of author and director, but as a model as well, was indeed an invitation to the dance.

COUNTDOWN TO SUCCESS

What I have learned is this: You are most likely to get into shape when you have an invitation, an impending event, a reason, a clock that is counting down to your success. Once you accept that invitation or choose your target, one of the hardest steps is indeed behind you. You must set and define a goal, or you will simply spin your wheels ad infinitum. Everyone has something to prove, not to others but to themselves.

Why is it critical that you act now? This is the single most important question that you can ask yourself. If you're like me, it's about more than just peaking for an event. It's about reclaiming "you." Just as in sitting through a bad movie when you can never get back those two precious lost hours, I had lost time. I had lost myself over a period of nearly two years, and I now consider it worth it because in the search to reclaim me, I discovered that I will never again allow myself to sit through a "bad movie."

Did you wake up one fine morning and peer into the mirror to find a person who had instantly transformed into someone you no longer recognized? No. You may have had that feeling, but yours was a slow and gradual transformation. Whatever the reason you attribute to your current shape—lack of gym time, fear, laziness, an overwhelming sense of not knowing where to start, a self-imposed negative thought process or sense of self-doubt, contentment or depression—whatever it was, you do not like the image currently staring back at you in the mirror. Through too many trips to the local fast food restaurants, too many selections from the aisles in the middle of the food store (processed foods), instead of smarter choices from the outer perimeter (whole foods), your current body composition has brought you to this point.

Whether it's a wedding, a reunion, a reinvention of self following a break-up, the birth of a child, New Year's resolution, injury, doctor's orders, an intervention or personal challenge or goal, whatever your reason, this book is written for you. This is your efficient and linear pathway toward peaking for your particular event or day and feeling good about it. You won't be rushed: you'll be able to breathe the whole time while taking the progressive steps to a new you until finally arriving at that day's door. This is your template, your plan, your recipe for success.

LET'S WORK TOGETHER

I have taken into consideration resources. Some of you have access to a gym, and some don't. Some of you may travel. And whether you have extra money each month after the bills are paid, or if you're saving every penny for your impending wedding, I've got you covered. My

approach is not intimidating but instead liberating. I do not encourage you to go on a near zero-carb or starvation diet. I will have no trainer or coach scream at you, severely restricting your calories and making it nearly impossible for you to get through your normal day, let alone one that calls for a resistance workout and cardio on top of it. My plan is easily incorporated into your current schedule; it isn't overwhelming and takes the worry and guesswork out of getting ready to look and feel your best for an event in a limited amount of time, whatever your body-type or current composition. No longer are you on your own. I am in the trenches with you, for I too was not blessed with a super-fast metabolism and have to work just as hard as the next person to peak my body. We are in this together. The bottom line: You're going to fit into your dress or that suit . . . and fit into it well.

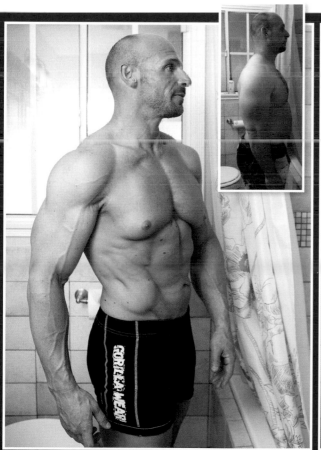

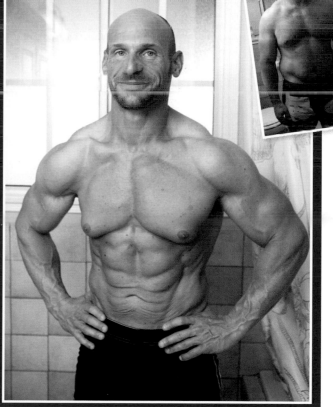

Mere weeks prior to my break-up I snapped a couple of pictures of myself to document just how far I had let my body go. There I was, tipping the scales at 246 pounds (112kg). I vowed that those two images (see insets) would be "before" photos and set out to uncover the real me. I began a fitness program and healthy diet that I dubbed my Peak Physique program, and stuck to it. Just months later, I stood in the same place to document my success, shooting these "after" photos that show a lean and fit me, weighing in at 197 pounds (89kg).

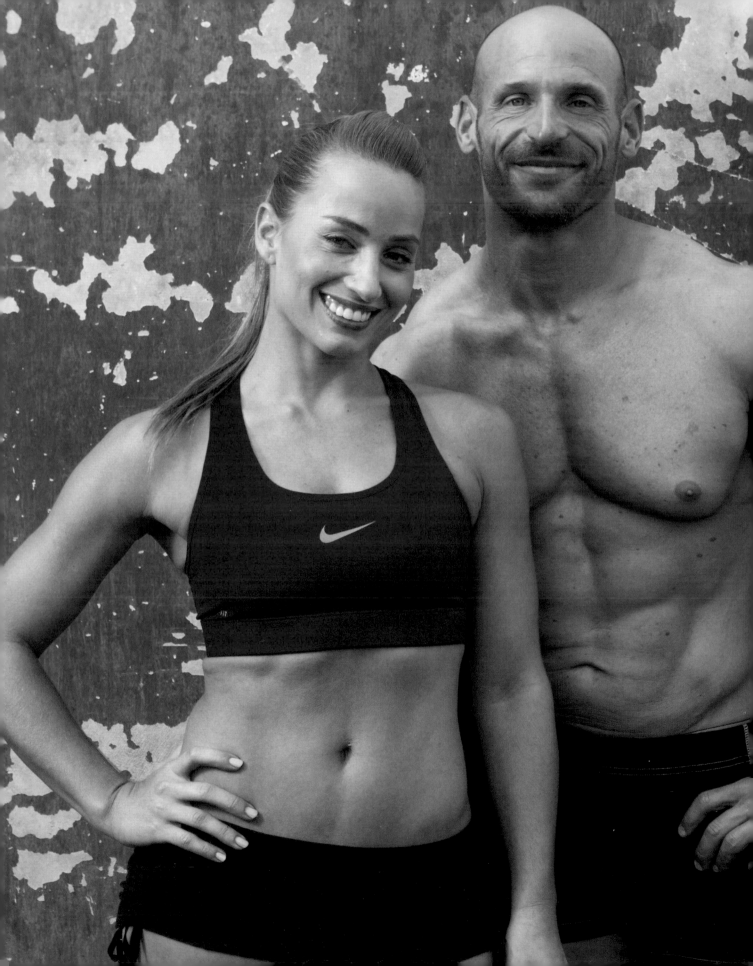

CHAPTER 1

PLAN OVERVIEW

Every great victory begins with an idea and then a mapped-out plan. Accomplishments are rarely achieved by accident, and, as such, the end result can seem overwhelming. But by systematically laying down a brick per day, eventually, a solid building will appear. Our basic, subconscious instinct as humans is to embrace pleasure and to avoid pain. This is at least partially why so many of us are apt to constantly cheat on our diets and take it easy in the gym or, in short, to consistently fail to achieve our physique goals.

But perhaps the plan was too restrictive in the first place: shooting for black belt status before even that white belt has been achieved. Since we can agree that the greatest pleasure will be your confident arrival at your event, we will fearlessly peer into the nucleus of pain together and progress through it linearly. Remember that while anyone can eat cheesecake, the taste of building your best body tastes infinitely better.

HOW WILL THIS BOOK HELP YOU?

Whatever your gender, shape and goal, your plan will consist of resistance training to hone and enhance the shape of your physique, cardiovascular activity to boost your metabolism and clean nutrition to leave you with minimal fat and maximal lean muscle mass. You, like the majority of people following this program, probably have fat to lose, not weight. Losing weight never results in just loss of body fat, but instead a mixture of muscle, fat and water. *No es bueno.*

It is safe to assume that if you're reading this, you're not hoping to gain weight going into your event and that is why the various protocols here are geared toward your two definitive goals: to lose body fat and hold onto precious muscle tissue. Losing weight isn't really all that difficult. You could restrict calories alone and would conceivably lose weight. Yet, you would appear deflated and soft instead of hard and firm, your body jettisoning muscle tissue in the process while retaining its fat stores. 1-800-NOT-WHAT-WE'RE-SHOOTING-FOR.

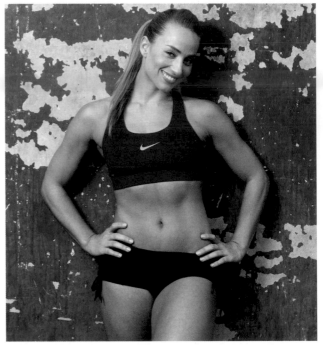

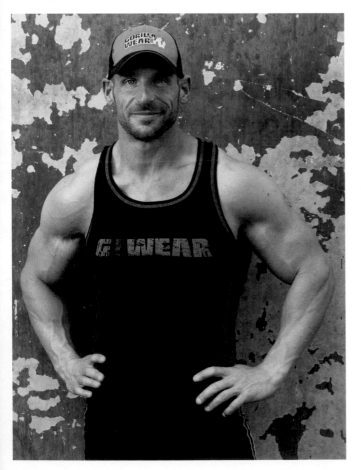

So how do you best use this book?

This program speaks to a mass audience. Although one size does not fit all (the artful independent movie, if you will, versus the blockbuster), there is something to be said of the Costco mass approach that definitely delivers. Your plan is not built on excessive training, marathon-like cardiovascular sessions or a tiny plate of food in a torturous, neglectful and monotonous Groundhog Day–like existence to punish you into results. Structure is in place in a time-managed, precise and stimulating program to provide maximum results in minimal time. Because both the male and female body have the same musculature and, for our purposes here, the same goals, the programs are nearly identical. The only difference will be in the recommended calorie intake, which is generally higher for a man because he tends to carry more lean tissue than a woman.

So how long is your program?

It has been my experience that noticeable results cannot be rushed and that changes begin to occur at around the 4-week mark, noticeable changes at around the 8-week mark, and serious stop-the-needle-on-a-record changes at the 12-week mark. Eventually, similar to when a woman is pregnant and the day comes when it is overwhelmingly obvious, so too will your body reflect dramatic positive change as you further get into shape.

Rather than feeling overwhelmed and committing to a full 12-week program, pick your target day months prior to it, and then have a go at it. Once you're on a roll and especially when people are complimenting you unsolicited, you'll find it hard to stop. Whether you take on this program for 4 weeks or 12, you can be assured that you'll be both looking and feeling better than you did on week 1. This is a win-win situation, one in which you cannot possibly lose.

So how do you apply this book?

Your exercise portion consists of three phases of training protocols that start with a minimum of activity and slowly intensify during each phase. The nutritional protocol offers suggested guidelines, dishes and sample menus in delivering five healthy and nutritious meals throughout your day to power you with energy and fuel for your workouts. It will also help you melt off body fat while showcasing lean muscles. Now, here's how you'll be resetting yourself

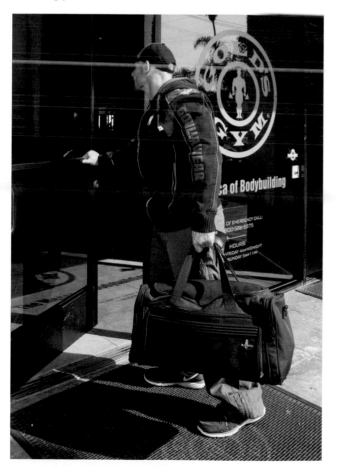

PROGRAM BREAKDOWN

PHASE 1: WEEKS 1–4
BEGINNER TRAINING PROTOCOL

Your instincts here might tell you this is not enough work. Pay no attention to such warnings and voices. During this initial phase of your training, you are learning proper sequencing of exercises, a consistent workload and how to properly fire from that particular day's workout and muscles used.

MONDAY	Chest/Back/Abdominals/30-Minute Cardio
TUESDAY	OFF
WEDNESDAY	Legs/30-Minute Cardio
THURSDAY	OFF
FRIDAY	Shoulders/Arms/Abdominals/30-Minute Cardio
SATURDAY	OFF
SUNDAY	OFF

PHASE 2: WEEKS 5–8
INTERMEDIATE TRAINING PROTOCOL

The inclusion of both a fourth day of cardio and a fourth day of resistance training allows you to give more individualized attention to each muscle group, as well as further speed up your metabolism for a true fat-incinerating state. In addition, for additional muscle detail and development, a few exercises and a third day of abdominals have been added. And you still have weekends off!

MONDAY	Chest/Triceps/Abdominals/30-Minute Cardio
TUESDAY	Back/30-Minute Cardio
WEDNESDAY	OFF
THURSDAY	Legs/Abdominals/30-Minute Cardio
FRIDAY	Shoulders/Biceps/Abdominals/30-Minute Cardio
SATURDAY	OFF
SUNDAY	OFF

PHASE 3: WEEKS 9–12
ADVANCED TRAINING PROTOCOL

The final phase of preparation, while still at four days of resistance training per week, has not only tacked on an extra day of cardio, but upped each day from 30 minutes to 40. This extra cardio will result in one thing: the additional shedding of unwanted body fat. For further overall development and tone, my all-time-favorite exercise, the deadlift has been added, along with a few arm-shaping exercises.

MONDAY	Chest/Triceps/Abdominals/40-Minute Cardio
TUESDAY	Back/40-Minute Cardio
WEDNESDAY	OFF
THURSDAY	Legs/Abdominals/40-Minute Cardio
FRIDAY	Shoulders/Biceps/Abdominals/40-Minute Cardio
SATURDAY	40-Minute Cardio
SUNDAY	OFF

REASONABLE GOALS = MAXIMUM GAINS

Whether you complete the physical work prior to your daily activities, during a lunch break or in the evening is entirely up to you. The most important factor is consistency. You are undertaking this journey, and your only competition is you. It is your mission to better the physique and self-image of the reflection that stares back at you in the mirror. You must do the best you can, and if you miss a day, make every effort to make it up at some point during your week. This plan need not be perfect but rather continual. Remember, not every hit will result in a home run.

Your goals need to be reasonable, not impossible. Quick-fix solutions and cramming simply do not work. Even fasting and extreme measures such as liposuction or powerful fat-burning thyroid drugs are not long-term solutions. Fasting often results in a rebound effect—once off the fast, you end up eating everything in sight. If you don't alter or curtail past negative associations with food following augmentation, the remaining fat cells will balloon and possibly multiply in size. Good-bye, bikini.

I've largely based the principles and methodologies of this book on what is the least amount that must be done in order to obtain the maximum outcome. It's all about efficiency, not the workload. This cannot be stressed enough: hours of cardio per day and a highly restrictive diet, along with excessive amounts of resistance, is not the way to go. Furthermore, this is why, for many of us, past attempts at getting into shape fail: we aim too high, too soon, and the plan is too unrealistic to maintain for long.

We are in this together for the long haul. Our goal is not to sprint to the finish line and collapse, but rather jog there, pause for reflection and carry on at a comfortable and attainable pace. Training is not about making one break, but rather overcoming your previous best. It's also not about how much weight you lift or how sore you may be. What matters most is keeping tension on the muscles during your working sets and not recruiting ancillary helpers.

BAD NEWS/GOOD NEWS

The bad news is that we have no control over the basic shape, or somatype, of our bodies. Each of us is born with

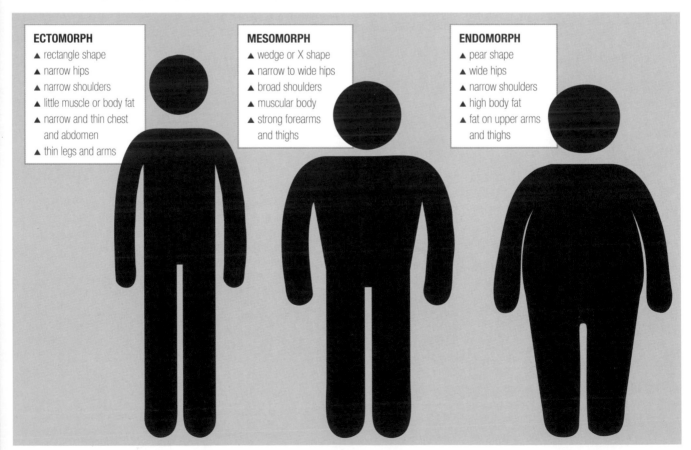

ECTOMORPH
- ▲ rectangle shape
- ▲ narrow hips
- ▲ narrow shoulders
- ▲ little muscle or body fat
- ▲ narrow and thin chest and abdomen
- ▲ thin legs and arms

MESOMORPH
- ▲ wedge or X shape
- ▲ narrow to wide hips
- ▲ broad shoulders
- ▲ muscular body
- ▲ strong forearms and thighs

ENDOMORPH
- ▲ pear shape
- ▲ wide hips
- ▲ narrow shoulders
- ▲ high body fat
- ▲ fat on upper arms and thighs

a genetic body type: Ectomorphs tend to have thin and lean bodies with speedy metabolisms. Endomorphs are prone to thick joints and midsections and can gain body fat rather easily. Mesomorphs are born with flattering X-frame structures, can gain lean muscle mass easily and keep fairly lean simultaneously. No one is purely one type—we are all a mixture leaning toward one dominant type. For the sake of your endeavors here, we can assume we're in the endomorphic category.

The good news is you absolutely have control over the quality of the composition of your body. If most of your body fat is stored in your trunk area and you have a wide waist, you can maximize your look by losing excess fat and accentuating your shoulders, which draws the eye away from less desirable areas. What cannot be accomplished is spot reduction or the voluntary riddance of body fat in one particular area. The body draws its fat stores from all over. Working your abs all day long will do little in the way of revealing newfound detail in your midsection. For example, the first place I tend to gain body fat is in my glutes, and it's always the last place it comes off. This is due to genetics. Yet, by working within "the rules," you essentially have complete control over your body!

YOUR ONE-STOP RESOURCE

This book is a general overview for getting you into shape. If you have special considerations such as diabetes, hyperextension, complications from giving birth or a host of other such important issues, please consult your physician or doctor before undertaking any kind of exercise and nutritional protocol. When your doctor has cleared you, and you have no contraindications, then this book is your one-stop resource.

Although the exercise sequences herein are precise, the given resistance is not, nor are the suggested nutritional guidelines suitable for everyone, because we are all different and at varying levels of fitness and actual body weights. What you can be assured of, however, is how to put all the legs together under one construct to properly sustain the table that is your body.

From here on out there will be no excuses. If you find you're low on time, you can exercise before or after work. Or on weekends. There is always time. If you're on a hectic travel schedule, I've also got you covered. You can workout in your hotel room if need be. All it takes is consistency plus my motto: Training + Cardio + Nutrition = Results.

This is the book that I would have loved to have had when I began working out all those years ago. This is the book that would have saved me years of trial and error,

frustration and sometimes false moves. This is the book that Jor-El should have secured in Kal-El's journey from Krypton to Earth, prior to him becoming Superman. These are more than words, for I am in the trenches with you. This is not a superior giving orders and watching from the safe confines of his office while his soldiers go to war. Trust me, I'm practicing what I preach, regularly. I even used the very principles and teachings within this book to achieve my own peak condition for the book's photo shoot.

The following pages contain the cumulative knowledge that I have learned, applied, refined and honed over the years and continue to utilize for great success with my clients, myself and now you. May it inspire, motivate and urge you to be the very best version of yourself that you can be. And for that, I dedicate this book to you, the reader, the practitioner, the go-getter and the achiever. Allow no one to get in your way—make them your way in.

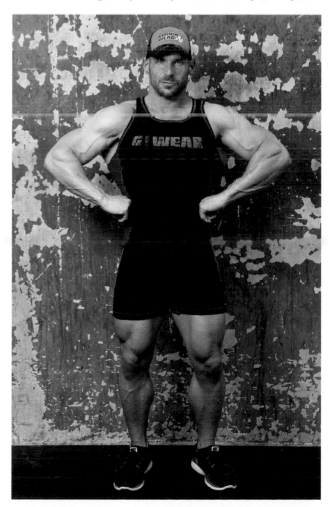

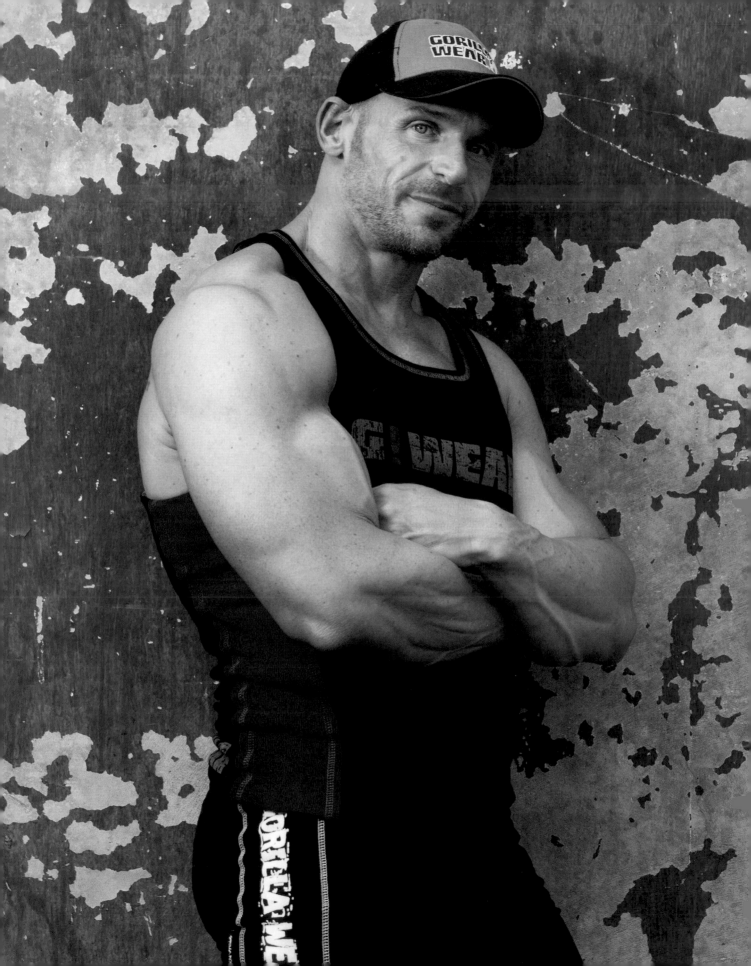

CHAPTER 2

MYTHS DEBUNKED, TRUISMS AND THE RULES OF THE GAME

Before undertaking any program or even digesting a syllabus, certain questions and concerns always come to mind. "Trust me" or "because" are, in my opinion, unacceptable answers to placate someone's need to know, no matter what your credentials are, especially when dealing with the body. This program is asking for many weeks of committed activity and nutrition on your part, so through logic, knowledge and progressive thinking, your concerns will be abated and your confidence at full capacity.

The following are some of the more common questions associated with getting into shape that I am routinely asked and their respective answers. Although some of these topics will come up in later chapters, let's set the record straight and tackle some common myths before Day 1 arrives.

Q I just want to lose weight fast and fit into my clothes. If I run a lot and eat very little, I can do it, right?

A This is a common myth and "strategy," and, most assuredly, it will head the pursuant toward disaster. Unlike a wrestler or boxer or other such athlete who must lose "weight" by doing an excessive amount of cardio wrapped in layers on a severely restricted eating regimen and is concerned solely with a number on a scale, here we are looking to lose body fat and retain lean muscle. We are focusing on a specific composition, not a general number. This process cannot be rushed or crammed for. Speeding for results is like shoveling too much snow in one scoop; eventually, you will give out and give up.

While cardiovascular activity is a part of the plan (to boost the metabolism), you should not perform it at too high an intensity. Overly high-intensive cardio, such as miles and miles of running, often just vacuums up excessive highly refined (sugar) calories, leaving you in a ravenous state. The result? Whatever has been burned has been replaced and then some. Yes, consuming fewer calories than are expended will result in weight loss, but that loss will come from muscle, water and fat and often leave you looking and feeling depleted. And the omission of resistance training will leave you mushy to the touch—not lean and firm. Eat to lose and lack of resistance is futile.

Q I am obsessed with the bathroom scale and check it daily for fluctuations in my weight. Isn't this a good thing?

A Numbers, are at best, only part of the big picture. It is the composition of the body that tells the true story. Your weight, especially if you are a woman, fluctuates daily. If you are concerned with numbers, have your body-fat composition taken or your blood-sugar levels checked if you are diabetic. For our endeavors here, this is a visual medium and as such, the mirror, photos and the way your clothes fit will reveal far more about your true condition than a number on your bathroom scale.

Q I'm concerned that weight training will make me big. A few sets of squats and my thighs get huge! And doesn't fat weigh more than muscle?

A Some people are just born lucky and respond to training more favorably than others will, but optimum muscle size is determined by genetic predisposition. Bulk is merely body fat covering muscle, giving the illusion of large, unflattering muscles. Some women who have a somewhat muscular appearance but who are not careful with their diet can develop this bulky appearance. By including weight training, upping their cardio activity and cleaning up their nutritional intake, they will be left with lean tissue—feeling and looking good.

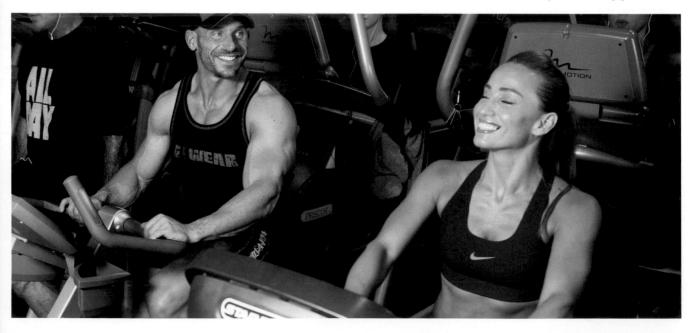

A pound of muscle weighs the same as a pound of fat, but muscle is more dense, taking up less space than fat. Fat will, however, take up more space or volume than muscle. To illustrate the point, think of two women, each the same height and weighing 150 pounds. One of them (let's call her "Subject A") has 19 percent body fat, while the other ("Subject B") has 35 percent. Do they look the same? Absolutely not—Subject A will look far better and be healthier than Subject B.

The more lean muscle mass you carry, the faster your metabolism runs in order to support that muscle. And keep in mind that muscle turning to fat if you stop training is another untruth. Muscle cells and fat cells are two different kinds of cells. We are born with a finite number of these cells. They simply increase or decrease in size over a lifetime (although if excessive weight is gained, the fat cells can further divide and multiply). If you cease training but eat clean, your muscle cells will simply shrink. If you consume junk, your fat cells will increase in size, causing you to gain unwanted body-fat.

In addition, many all-too-common surgeries can be avoided and ruled out with a lifestyle that includes regular weight training. I'll take a set of reverse hyperextensions over back surgery any day.

Q Time is a factor, and I always do my cardio first and then my weights, but I notice my energy is very low after the cardio. What am I doing wrong?

A Cardiovascular activity (motion without stopping for at least 20 minutes involving the heart) runs on adipose, or fat, for fuel. Anaerobic activity (stop-and-go motion such as weight training) runs on glycogen (stored carbohydrates). The function of cardio here, aside from supporting a healthy heart, is not to burn calories but rather to raise the metabolism. Calories burned are always replaced during the next meal. A metabolism that is fueled by small clean meals throughout the day will be efficient at burning body fat and holding onto precious muscle tissue.

The decision to implement cardio first followed by resistance training will result in you being tired at the start of resistance training largely because cardio depletes you. You are now asking your muscles to fire during resistance training when they are running on fumes. Always perform weight exercises first and then cardio—this way you will have the right fuel burning at the right time for the right activity.

It has been shown that cardio is highly effective first thing in the morning on an empty stomach and resistance training later in the day (following a meal). For many, these time parameters are unrealistic, so ideally stick with a light 5-minute cardio warm-up followed by resistance training and cardio, and then conclude with some form of stretching or myofascial release. If you're absolutely pressed for time, performing either an intense resistance-training workout with little rest in between sets or a full-body workout as demonstrated in chapter 6 is a superb alternative. Conversely, you won't speed up your results by spending more time in the gym. You can train short and intense or long and not intense. I don't know about you, but I'd rather face the music, do what has to be done efficiently and spend the rest of my day out of the gym.

Q I want abs, a strong core, a flat stomach and a six-pack now. All I do is work my abs until I'm blue in the face. Nothing is happening. Help! What do I do?

A The truth about your abs is this: they are worked from almost every exercise you could possibly perform. If you want your abdominals to be prominently displayed, your body-fat levels must be appropriately low.

A lot of direct abdominal work will make them stronger and even improve athletic performance, but a clean nutritional intake, cardio and resistance training will always be the best way to bring about abdominal definition—unless of course you're one of those people who can conceivably eat whatever they want and showcase abs year round. If you're holding this book in your hands, chances are you're not this person, and neither am I. This myth is also known as spot reduction. Theoretically you could be elated with most of your body except one spot, and even if you focused all of your will with a renewed ferocity on that one body part, fat will still be drawn most probably from someplace else, at least initially.

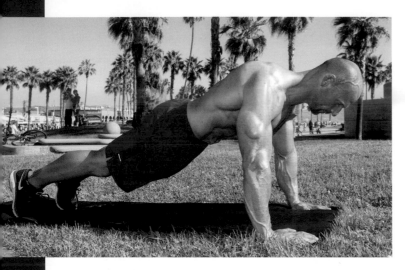

Q I'm totally with you and on board, it's just that my partner does not follow this lifestyle. What should I do?

A The best that you can. This is *your* journey: this is about *you*. Your partner, husband or wife need not be a fellow practitioner (though it would be nice), but should at least be supportive of your efforts. And maybe, just maybe, as you get closer to achieving your goals, he or she may join you. It's difficult to not pay attention to or mimic someone who's achieving. In any case, you have a job to do each day and no one will have your back more than you.

Q I do cardio, so I don't need to work my legs, and I have breasts, so I don't need to train my chest. Right?

A Everyone needs cardio for the heart and to help keep off unwanted body fat, but it's not enough. Resistance training for the legs is not only cardiovascular by nature, it also works your upper body (core-stabilizer and upper-body ancillary muscles) at the same time. That and to keep from looking like a light bulb (think symmetry) has always been enough to get me to duck under the squat bar.

Yes ladies, breast tissue is primarily fat tissue, but underneath it are your pectoral muscles, whose function is to draw the arm across the front of the body. Low body-fat levels will result in smaller breasts, but regular chest training will act as a push-pull. Your pecs will work along with your back muscles to keep you balanced and your posture in check. Good posture and less lower-back pain sounds good to me.

Q I don't like squats and am perfectly content to do the inner/outer thigh machines. Aren't they just as effective?

A The adductor-abductor machines are like walking to a store whereas squats are like driving— much more efficient. Yes, squats are difficult. After all, they make us feel as if we are being drilled into the ground. But they work most of the leg musculature as well as the core and are fantastic overall for your cardiovascular system. You can do your inner/outer thigh machines following squats, but they are to the legs what frosting is to cake.

Q I really want to improve my body-weight exercises so I have been doing push-ups, pull-ups and dips every day. But I'm not getting any stronger. In fact, I feel tired and weak. What should I do?

A A muscle can only grow stronger when consistently overloaded on a regular basis with good nutrition and adequate rest. Training something every day to improve it sounds good in theory, but in reality you are not allowing the muscle to recuperate. It is during rest that muscles recover and grow both bigger and stronger. This constant state of overtraining will not only result in weaker muscles, but could also cause them to tear or rip.

Q Low reps or high reps?

A Certain body parts, such as the legs, respond best to higher repetitions (12 to 15) and the upper body to lower reps (8 to 10). It is a myth that high reps will lean you out or help you to get ripped quicker. In actuality, higher reps with lighter weights are like taking the nails out of a house, thus weakening its structure. For a quality physique you must continue doing what brought you to the dance in the first place. Use the correct amount of repetitions to build muscle and your cardio and nutrition to best showcase it.

Q What is your opinion of CrossFit?

A I am not well versed on CrossFit, but many of my friends and colleagues are into it, and they look great. Nonetheless, I don't like anything with speed or momentum—couple that with overtraining and you're going to get hurt. I've built my physique and that of my countless students and clients over the years with the same tools: free weights, cardio, good nutrition, tension on the muscles, and slow and controlled repetitions. Of course I do believe there is more than one way to achieve a goal, and if CrossFit is it for you, go for it.

Q Do you do this stuff too? How do you really train?

A Yes, I do the same components week in and week out that I am prescribing for you. The key is knowing that you can't nor shouldn't floor the pedal all the time; sometimes you must coast or let up on the gas a little bit. Regardless, I believe in training each body part once per week only, and not twice. I believe in avoiding pleasure in the gym by making a given set easier, and I believe in embracing good pain or the stress of a workload on muscles. I believe in efficiency, not rushing, and I believe in safety. I also believe that many gym accidents begin outside of the gym whereby the hammer of a gun is often cocked by a sudden jerk, and in the gym the bullet is often fired. Gym accidents usually begin outside of the training arena.

Q I just want to be skinny! Why do I need to spend all this time in the gym? Can't I just go on a diet?

A Success in the gym starts with changing your thought patterns. "Skinny" and "thin" imply an emaciated look that is very unhealthy. "Lean and toned" sounds much better. For many of us, the road to success starts in the way we perceive things. We all have to cross a path, put in the time and work on a consistent basis in order to achieve. You need not fall in love with the process, but being passionate about putting forth the effort and trusting the process will pay huge dividends. *Diet* contains the word *die*, which is finite and short-lived. Replace it with the word *lifestyle*, implying "long-term," and this is how you do it, for life.

Q Isn't diet 90 percent of the game?

A To imply that diet equates to 90 percent of your results, and that all it takes is a paltry 10 percent in the gym is ludicrous. Training, nutrition and cardio

are all important in garnering you results. I will say, though, that the leaner you become or as you get closer to achieving peak condition, the more important diet can become.

Q How do I go to a party and not overeat or drink?

A This is probably the number-one question that I am asked during the holiday season. Because we all indulge from time to time, either join the party for one sumptuous meal on this special occasion or think and plan ahead for the big day. Sometimes I will have a small healthy meal just as I arrive at a party to keep myself satiated. Although eating clean at a party can be difficult, it's not impossible. Look for leaner food choices. Perhaps cold cuts like turkey breast or roast beef, whole wheat bread, raw nuts and some vegetables. Just watch out for the dip. A diet soda or even a glass of wine or light beer won't hamper your efforts.

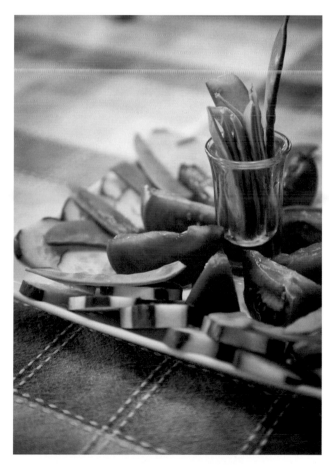

THE RULES OF THE GAME

What follows are some of my favorite and most effective training principles to help you along with the workout portion of the program.

Target sets

Warm-up sets and working sets are the two types of sets we are concerned with. As a car goes from 20 to 60 miles per hour, so too must your body work up from a lighter resistance to a progressively heavier one during the course of your workout. Lifting the same resistance on consecutive sets is both inefficient and a waste of time. Progress can be achieved by striving for an extra repetition or a slightly heavier weight on the last or main set of a given exercise. Stay fully focused during your workouts, and give the most to your working (main) sets. I believe the more experience you have in the gym, the fewer overall sets you will need, for you are able to generate a level of intensity that a beginner is not yet capable of.

This principle has always been the cornerstone of my training. Think of a carpenter with a hammer and nail. An inexperienced carpenter needs to take numerous swings or whacks with the hammer to drive the nail into the wood. This is not only time-consuming and inefficient but risks damaging the wood. An experienced carpenter, however, will hit the nail in with one or two swings to efficiently and accurately get the job done. The more training experience you have, the more you can get out a given set of an exercise. If you're only performing a few working sets for each exercise, you're going to want to give your all to each and every set and make them count.

Tension on the muscle

The name of the game is to stimulate, not annihilate. You are in the gym to efficiently target that particular day's target muscles. It's human nature to want to breeze

through a set and recruit other muscle groups when the burn becomes too intense. To keep your focus on the right muscles, try the rest/pause technique, which calls for you to put a weight down just before your form gets too sloppy during a set. Wait a few seconds, and then complete a few more clean repetitions. The result will be improvements to your physique as well as fewer injuries and more longevity for your body.

Rest

Rushing through your workout will do little to maximize the effectiveness of your program and can actually be counterproductive. Forget about the person next to you sweating profusely, bouncing about the gym like a human pinball and full of excessive pre-workout stimulants, going from exercise to exercise and using more swing and momentum than muscle and control. Take as long as you need to rest between sets to give your all. Certain movements like squats will require more rest than say a smaller movement such as barbell curls. Take your time.

Function

One of the great things about this program is that it's all planned out for you. As a personal trainer, I am sometimes asked if I make up the routines on the spot and how do I put things together? To me exercise routines are like professional wrestling matches. Know the beginning and ending and how to connect the two points by an educated improvisation. Be firm, yet malleable. For exercise selections, knowing the function of a muscle is a key and clear indicator of what needs to be done. The pectorals, for example, are responsible for drawing the arm across the torso and so, at some point in the workout, a flye movement needs to be incorporated.

Adaptability

Because your primary goal here is losing fat and holding onto lean muscle tissue, ancillary wants such as maximum strength and minutes shaved off your best performance times are off your radar screen . . . but not entirely. Part of the fun and allure of this program is seeing and feeling the weekly changes within your body as that newly lean person comes out of its shell. As our bodies adapt to exercise, the changes to them come more slowly. By the law of diminishing returns, a neophyte who has not worked out before or someone who's avoided the gym for a long while will progress more rapidly than someone who is regularly at it. To prevent stagnation and boredom, keep track of your best lifts and body-fat percentage.

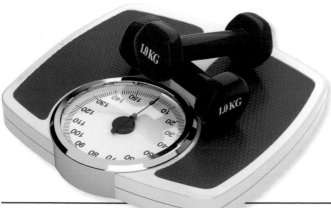

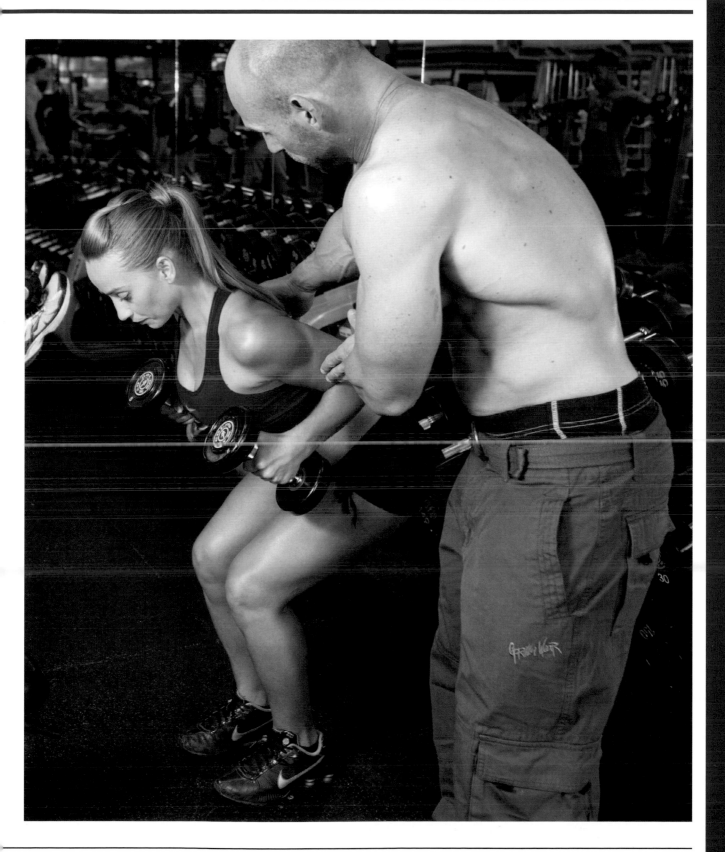

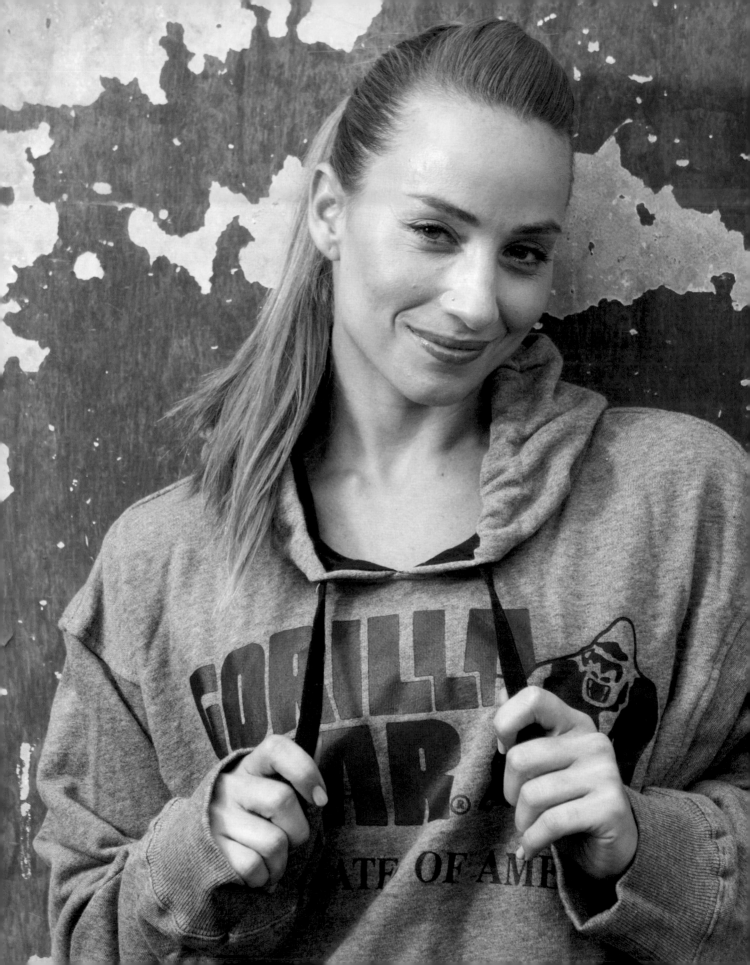

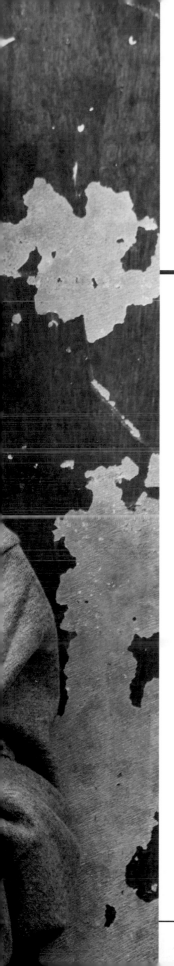

CHAPTER 3

THE MENTAL EDGE

If you've bought this book, signed up for the gym membership, thrown out the junk food and yet still feel like starting next week, or a few weeks after that . . . then you need to refine, redefine, reexamine and reorganize your mental processes, before we can even begin to tackle the physical.

Motivation, the mental behind the physical, the wizard behind the curtain if you will, is so important, so all-encompassing, that it needs nothing less than its own chapter. The body cannot perform without the brain. If you're programmed for success and focused, very little can stop you. You can begin to get your body in order by taking the lead with your mind.

DON'T GET DERAILED

For some people, motivation is a given. Assign them a task or goal and they set forth, take a step every day and wind up like clockwork at the finish line. For many of us, although we can target a specific and defined goal, we put it off by saying we'll start the next week. Next week turns into next month—if and when we finally start. And often, after many false starts and attempts, we simply abort the mission, deeming it—if we're able to admit—too far out of our reach, too hard and unobtainable.

But why the derailment? Some may lack a plan, some the will and others the fortitude to cross a given bridge. But a goal without motivation is like an actor reading some lines. Lacking the motivation, we don't know where the character is coming from or what they are capable of. But arm the actor with a motivation or an "I wish to" statement, and suddenly those words leap off the page and are given life and meaning.

We all know that anything really worth attaining in life takes hard work. The mental anguish in putting off hard work often takes more of a toll on us than the actual work itself. So if we can eliminate the fear of hard work, or at least face it, then a large part of the mental battle is overcome.

CONTINUANCE

Motivation can come from many sources, and we all need sustained motivation for the most important part of our journey—continuance. For there are those days when waking up extra early to complete your workout for the day results in oversleeping, or when the gym is near empty, and you can't readily feed off the energy and looks from others. And then there are those evenings, after a long workday, when the last thing you can possibly imagine doing is ducking under a squat bar. To this I say: always do the best you can. Again, not every hit results in a home run. If you miss a day, do your best to get back on track and pick up right where you left off. Don't allow a glitch early in the week to erase the potential progress of the rest of the week. Don't wait to start anew the following Monday. The key is to get right back on the horse following a missed workout or a cheat meal.

I've had many Fridays jam-packed with work and filled with items that need my immediate attention, so I make a deal with myself that I'll head to the gym right after breakfast Saturday morning, and then I can get on with my weekend. And I keep to that deal.

If you're not yet looking the way you want to, put yourself in the danger zone by making yourself accountable. How can you best do that?

Believe it or not, committing yourself to an event or endeavor in which you must show up at your best is an excellent way to program yourself for long-term motivation. For example, during my days as a competitive bodybuilder, I had no choice but to stay motivated to work out and look my best at all times. I had committed myself to the sport. I had four main reasons for keeping that commitment: I would be posing basically in nothing but my underwear in front of hundreds of people; my parents were paying for all of my chicken breast protein needs, and in their love and investment I could not let them down. I gave my word I would compete, and I was consumed with seeing how far I could take my physique. In my case, my 12-week commitment resulted in a big win and a national title . . . many chicken breasts later.

Don't subscribe to a super-strict and unrealistic program that starts Monday and ends Wednesday only to be resumed next Monday, as if Monday is some magical beginning point. Instead, ask yourself, "Why am I doing this?" As I shared earlier, in my own case, a very painful breakup had left me many fat pounds above where I needed to be. I decided to reinvent myself, and along the way the reinvention led to the creation of this book. So start imperfectly, eliminate the nonessential or less important items and get on board. Your thread, spine or reason already exists. It's why you have this book in your hands now. If you live more of your Sundays with the work ethic of a Monday, you *will* succeed. Follow your program with a sense of urgency and you will succeed.

THE TOP 10

It is my duty to instill and reemphasize that no matter the current state of your affairs, your body is your most valuable asset. And you absolutely have control over changing your physique for the better at any age and circumstance. I believe that motivation is the vein to your heart—your heart being your goal. What follows, in no particular order, are my top 10 motivationalisms. They are all important, doable reminders that will see your journey through to successful completion.

1. The Big O

It's "O" as in "occasion." Wedding, bar mitzvah, reunion or some other occasion coming up? Goal setting is always more in the here and now when you introduce a time frame. This is the catalyst needed to get you going, to get you invested. Once you have an occasion and a date, coupled with the means (the tools) and the will (you), nothing can stop you.

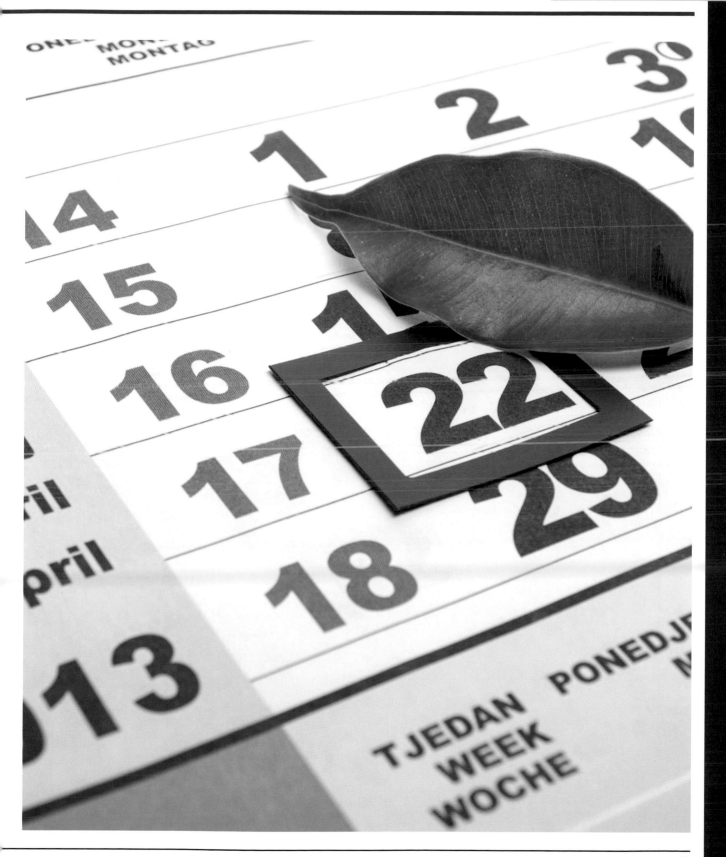

AUGUST

AOÛT ▲ AGOSTO ▲ AUGUST

	MONDAY Lun Lun Mon	**TUESDAY** Mar Mar Die	**WEDNESDAY** Mer Miér Mit	**THURSDAY** Jeu Jue Don	**FRIDAY** Ven Vier Fre	**SATURDAY** Sam Sáb Sam	**SUNDAY** Dim Dom Son
WEEK 8		1 Back/ 30-Minute Cardio X	2 OFF X	3 Legs/ Abdominals/ 30-Minute Cardio X	4 Shoulders/ Biceps/ Abdominals/ 30-Minute Cardio X	5 OFF X	6 OFF X
WEEK 9	7 Chest/Triceps/ Abdominals/ 40-Minute Cardio X	8 Back/ 40-Minute Cardio X	9 OFF X	10 Legs/ Abdominals/ 40-Minute Cardio X	11 Shoulders/ Biceps/ Abdominals/ 40-Minute Cardio X	12 40-Minute Cardio X	13 OFF X
WEEK 10	14 Chest/ Triceps/ Abdominals/ 40-Minute Cardio X	15 Back/ 40-Minute Cardio C	16 OFF (Make up for cheat meal!) X	17 Legs/ Abdominals/ 40-Minute Cardio X	18 Shoulders/ Biceps/ Abdominals/ 40-Minute Cardio X	19 40-Minute Cardio X	20 OFF X
WEEK 11	21 Chest/ Triceps/ Abdominals/ 40-Minute Cardio X	22 Back/ 40-Minute Cardio X	23 OFF	24 Legs/ Abdominals/ 40-Minute Cardio	25 Shoulders/ Biceps/ Abdominals/ 40-Minute Cardio	26 40-Minute Cardio	27 OFF
WEEK 12	28 Chest/ Triceps/ Abdominals/ 40-Minute Cardio	29 Back/ 40-Minute Cardio	30 OFF	31 Legs/ Abdominals/ 40-Minute Cardio	1 Shoulders/ Biceps/ Abdominals/ 40-Minute Cardio	2 40-Minute Cardio	3 Reunion!!

2. Calendar

Use a single sheet of paper, showing one month at a time. Draw an X for each healthy day of eating and training and a big C for a cheat meal or blemish. At the end of the countdown to the big event, you should see a lot more Xs.

3. Validation

To be validated is to be heard, valued and seen, and it is indeed a powerful tool. Posting update pictures on Facebook and other social media sites is a good way to get support from others when you sometimes lack continuance of the journey. Contrary to validation are those who will be jealous, skeptical or quite simply can't identify with your current goals. If anyone doubts you to the point of questioning you or ridiculing you, get that person out of your life. There's enough negativity in the world, and your workout should be your sanctuary and your time for bettering you.

4. Picture

Our journey is mainly a visual one and starts with a picture of you, right now—as unflattering as that may be. Take a photo and put it away. Then, find a picture of someone's body that you aspire to have and tape it to your fridge, make it the wallpaper on your phone, or display it anywhere you can view it daily. You could even post a picture or invitation of your upcoming event for definitive inspiration and a locked-in "I'm attending" attitude.

5. If the shoe doesn't fit, make it

Find a piece of clothing that once fitted, but is now less than flattering or a new garment that you would love to wear for the big event. Your goal is to make it fit and fit well. Not in 2 weeks but rather in a slow 12-week fat-melting campaign.

6. Tell everyone

The people close to you care and will support you in your quest to achieve your goals and aspirations. I guarantee that they will not only keep tabs on your progress, but that you might also even motivate them to make the shoe fit once again in their own lives.

7. Maintain the course

No one gets out of shape in a week and neither can they get fit again in the same amount of time. Aiming for 1 to 2 pounds of fat loss per week adds up to dozens of pounds of fat over the course of just a few short months. Patience, commitment and diligence are among the weapons in your arsenal. In addition, your instincts play a vital role in your success. Years ago, as I was getting ready for my first physique contest, a few weeks before the show a fellow competitor questioned why I was still using relatively heavy weights. Although this was my first competition and I was inexperienced, I reasoned that training light up to the event would cause me to lose precious muscle tissue. I further mentioned that I must continue to do what brought my physique this far in the first place. He dismissed me and a few weeks later, his placing was dismissive. I won my class. Instincts: trust them.

8. Good-bye

Jettison unhealthy foods. Get rid of all of it, *now*. All garbage foods and empty calories in the bin. If you are having a split decision or instinctive urge to cheat, you now have to get dressed to do so. Or at least put on underwear and hit the drive-thru. I'm in favor of the occasional cheat meal, just don't make it too easy or too often.

9. Ancillary recruits

Bringing in a personal trainer or any other such unbiased professional will not only help to keep you motivated, it will also get you to your goals faster. You are looking to make long-distance positive changes to your lifestyle, not short-term, sprint-style temporary fixes. When in doubt, see a fitness professional whose job it is to regularly get clients to fit into new, flattering shoes.

10. Check in

Regularly attempt to put that shoe on. It may not yet fit, but in the weeks to follow, you will wedge in a toe, and that, my friend, is progress.

BURN WITH A MAGNIFICENT CONSISTENT MADNESS!

Here is one last story on motivation. A few years ago a friend had come to Los Angeles to visit and see the sights. I hadn't seen her in some time, and she was, admittedly, out of shape. At our first destination, there was an escalator and a flight of stairs. She challenged me to race up the stairs. I declined and took the escalator to enjoy the sights and sounds of the beautiful structure surrounding us. I had no sense of competition. The war was only within myself and only to take place during my workout. She skipped, jumped and hightailed it to the top only to "beat me" and arrived short of breath, hunched over and inhaling rapidly. I patted her on the back, and said, "When you can focus on a less brightly lit fire that burns steadily and consistently, then and only then will you truly win."

It's not about a short and intense effort, but rather a long-distance non-rushed continued journey.

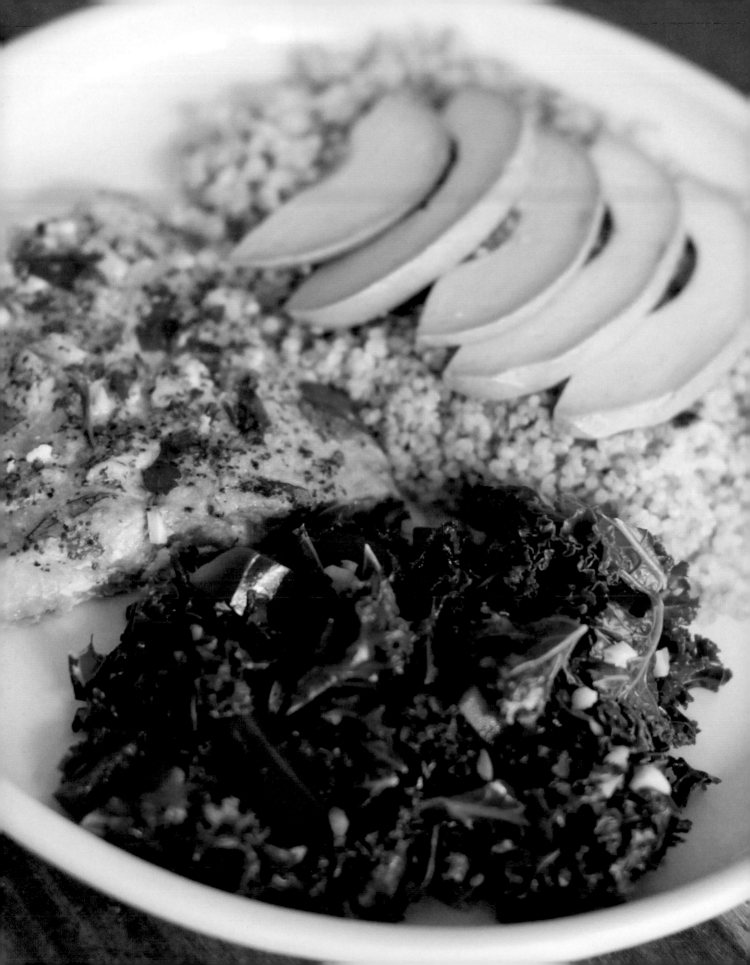

CHAPTER 4

THE FUEL

The subject of nutrition and its relation to the body is a subjective topic open to countless interpretations. There's a near-infinite industry that includes books, suggested food groups, charts, courses and even phone apps. Carbs? No carbs? Fat is good. Fat is bad. Eat breakfast. Skip breakfast.

What we can agree on is that food is fuel. What we consume is essentially what we wear on the outside, how we feel on the inside and what allows us to perform activities as varied as turning a key in a lock to running on an open stretch of road. Without fuel there is no life.

FOOD: NOT JUST ABOUT NUTRITION

Food is, for many, the centerpiece of celebration. We eat when we are joyous and happy with family and friends during some of life's finest moments. We are rewarded with food, we turn to food when we are happy, sad, nervous and anxious. We're told as youths we must eat the basics to survive. We are shown charts, served largely unhealthy foods in school and then left to our own devices. When we grow into adults, some of us develop diseases such as diabetes and rather than fix the actual problem (poor diet), we at best put a band-aid over cancer with prescription drug after drug for life.

For our purposes here, the mission is to arm you with the proper knowledge of how to best fuel yourself both at home and out in the world for fat loss, lean muscle occurrence and to function and feel good in life. Anyone can become skinny or thin by simply reducing one's caloric intake, but the result will be a weak, emaciated and temporary state that often rebounds in an excessive weight gain following the reintroduction of excess, refined macronutrients.

EAT TO LOSE

Yesteryear's approach of a breakfast, lunch and dinner is quite simply not enough fuel to properly propel the machine that is you, especially with your weekly workouts. You must eat to lose. Banish thoughts of severe caloric restriction and skipping breakfast or ridiculous notions such as no carbs after a certain time. These practices are too extreme and demanding and almost always result in excessively cheating on your diet and constantly thwarting your progress.

Take, for example, the notion of skipping breakfast and instead having a sugared-coffee concoction. Not only will you begin your day without much needed long-term energy, you're also sure to crash for a lack of it. Having poor nutrition instead of real nutrition is like driving with only one gallon of gas in the tank. Once that gallon is used up, the remaining fumes will only carry you so far. And if you're lucky, into the next fueling station.

Not having complex carbohydrates after a certain time in the afternoon usually results in an overindulgence of them much later in the evening when you don't need them, i.e., when resting or sleeping. Think of meals as bridge points. Small frequently placed pillars spread across the span will support the structure (body), whereas too few points results in a weakened, unsupported state.

The concept of eating to lose is a critical one to learn and apply. Many people will limit not only the frequency of their meals but also the calories (a stored unit of energy) and nutrients contained therein. As discussed, breakfast is often omitted in favor of a highly processed sugary coffee. Lunch is light on sufficient clean fuel, usually consisting of a processed food such as bread and minimal protein served with condiments that are high in saturated fat. Dinner is an overboard extravaganza that leaves the perpetrator full, restless, guilt-ridden the next day and, what's worse, higher in both body fat and body weight. And then the whole starvation cycle begins anew the following morning.

ON THE ESSENTIALS

Your resting energy expenditure is the total number of calories needed to exist. Your total daily energy expenditure is the total number of calories needed for existence plus your total number of calories used for daily physical activity as well as for digestion. In order to lose body fat you must take in fewer calories than expended, and utilize stored calories in the form of fat during exercise. The key of course is to avoid burning muscle tissue as fuel.

Nutritional success begins with an understanding that multiple (4 to 5) daily meals, which are unprocessed (consumed in an natural state) and contain a balance of macronutrients, spread throughout the day will help your body to utilize stored adipose (fat) as fuel. These macronutrients, protein (muscle mass, 4 calories per gram), carbohydrates (energy, 4 calories per gram) and fats (joint lubrication, protection of the heart, 9 calories per gram) are the mainstays of the nutritional skeleton if you will.

Furthermore, the macronutrients are the important numbers we need be concerned with versus calories. For example, an 8-oz (225g) raw, skinless chicken breast contains roughly 250 calories, but what are those calories composed of? Further exploration into the macronutrients tells us this food contains roughly 50 grams of protein, 3 grams of fat and 0 grams of carbohydrates. This is a much bigger reveal of what is actually going into our bodies beyond just calories alone.

Here's the most important paragraph in this chapter: Insulin is a hormone that drives fat storage. The key is to avoid foods that spike insulin levels, such as many high-glycemic carbohydrates and processed foods, which are high in sugar. These trigger insulin production, and the insulin can then store the calories as fat. Carbohydrates are essentially sugars, and as such they are broken down into glucose and absorbed directly into the bloodstream during digestion and they can spike insulin levels. Proteins and fats do little as far as spiking insulin levels, and that is why it is important to include them in your meals. Furthermore, while a potato (a carbohydrate) alone will spike levels, when combined with a protein, fat and leafy green, the result is a slower rate of digestion as well as a lower insulin release by the body and, ultimately, less fat storage. Although excess calories beyond body maintenance can be stored as fat, processed carbohydrates have a much higher tendency over protein and even fats.

Know that good nutrition is at least as important as your training and the two are synergistic. When properly combined, you can be assured to make the absolute most of your physique. In essence, eating as our ancestors did, with a diet of proteins, fats, leafy green vegetables and naturally occurring carbohydrates, will not only help to keep you fueled, it will also keep your body lean. Our ancestors also moved and lifted constantly in order to locate and harvest their fuel.

PREMIUM OPTIONS

Here is a general overview of some of the very best foods to fuel you and help to keep you lean.

Proteins:

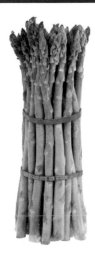

- egg whites (one yolk for every three whites)
- chicken breast
- turkey breast
- most fish
- top-round or rump steak
- low-fat cottage cheese
- low-sugar Greek yogurt
- RTD (ready-to-drink protein shakes)

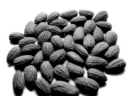

Fats:

- fish oil
- flax seed oil
- avocado
- raw nuts

Carbohydrates (complex):

- beans
- brown rice
- quinoa
- oatmeal (porridge)
- yams/sweet potatoes
- sprouted grain/whole-grain bread

Carbohydrates (fibrous):

- broccoli
- asparagus
- brussels sprouts
- salad

Drinks:

- water
- unsweetened iced tea
- black coffee
- diet soda/sugar-free drinks

THE GLYCEMIC INDEX

If the majority of your intake is composed of food from the Premium Options lists, you're well on your way toward achieving a long-term lean body. Further smart choices can be found by looking at the Glycemic Index (GI).

The Glycemic Index can help you track your carbohydrate intake, allowing you to gauge whether you are eating "good" or "bad" carbs. We now know that not only are all carbohydrates not "bad," but they are also not equal to one another in terms of insulin release and fat storage. The GI tells us how quickly our blood-sugar levels rise after consuming certain kinds of carbohydrates. It is through the proper use and adherence to this measure that maintaining a long-term lean body is both realistic and possible.

Look for carbohydrates with low GI scores ranking 55 or lower, and avoid those with high scores. White bread, white potatoes, white rice and alcoholic drinks have high GI score ratings of 70 or above. Medium-GI choices include croissants, muffins, pizza and shredded wheat, rating 56 to 69. Low-GI foods include lentils, legumes, nuts and most vegetables, with scores of 55 or lower.

Limit:

- most dairy
- high-glycemic fruit
- soda
- juice
- alcohol
- bread and cereal
- pasta
- butter
- margarine
- heavy oil
- fried food

PREMIUM REPLACEMENTS

Although you may have to limit or avoid certain foods, you don't have to give up flavor or variety. There are plenty of easy substitutions you can make that allow you to indulge while stile staying on target.

- Replace low-fat peanut butter with regular peanut butter. The bit of fat you're saving has been replaced with sugar, and that equals more stored fat on your body.
- Replace heavy condiments with spices. Most condiments are high in sugar. Spices are not only calorie-free but they also add a lot of zest and flavor to an otherwise healthy but bland meal. Additionally, the spicier the better, because this can help to produce a thermogenic effect within your body and help to raise your metabolism.
- Replace ground turkey meat, which contains not just white meat but also dark meat and skin and who knows what else (and is often more fattening than hamburger) with lean ground turkey breast. Take a minute to read the label.

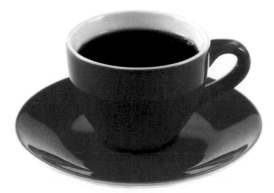

- Replace bananas, raisins and pineapple with berries, grapefruit or apples. In moderation, of course, the latter three are lower on the Glycemic Index and thus register less in raising blood glucose levels.
- Replace juice with water and lemon. Would you ever consume 10 oranges in one sitting? No, but you could easily drink that many in a glass of juice. Lots of extra sugar versus calorie-free nourishment plus vitamin C.
- Replace energy drinks with black coffee or tea. Sugar, sugar and more sugar combined with caffeine versus near calorie-free caffeine.

- Replace regular yogurt with low-fat/low-sugar Greek-style yogurt. Super high in sugar (nearly all of its carbs) versus this super-high protein/low-sugar alternative.
- Replace alcohol with diet soda or a sugar-free drink. Vodka, wine or what have you, alcohol is alcohol and is seven useless calories per gram versus diet soda clocking in at zero calories (in moderation of course).
- Replace most boxed cereals with oatmeal/porridge. Keep in mind that refined carbs = sugar = non-sustained energy versus sustained "clean" energy.
- Replace mayonnaise with spicy mustard for tuna fish. Your palate will indeed be satisfied while you avoid all the extra fat.

FILLING YOUR SHOPPING CART

Here is a list of foods I fill my basket with for my complete nutritional support. As a general rule, when food shopping, spend less time wandering up and down the middle aisles, where the foods are highly processed, and stick mostly to the outer perimeters of the store, where foods are fresh and in their raw, unprocessed state. And never shop when you are hungry—you'll be too tempted to make poor choices.

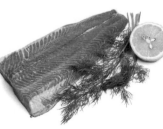

- water
- diet ginger ale
- diet cola
- tea
- coffee
- brussels sprouts
- yams/sweet potatoes
- asparagus
- lettuce
- garbanzo beans/chickpeas
- raw almonds
- raw almond butter
- turkey breast filets
- ground turkey breast
- chicken breasts
- wild-caught salmon
- frozen tilapia, sea bass
- frozen cod
- tuna canned and packed in water
- lean ground beef (4 percent fat)

- oats/porridge
- quinoa, unprepared
- ready-made quinoa bowl
- brown rice, unprepared
- ready-made brown rice bowl
- Thai jasmine rice
- brown rice and beans in a can
- wholemeal bread
- low-fat Greek yogurt
- eggs
- garlic powder
- calorie-free sweetener
- Cajun spice
- cinnamon
- habanero hot sauce
- hot salsa

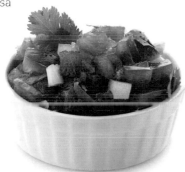

Although it would be difficult to provide an example of daily nutrition for every particular body type and weight, because we all are different, what you can take away from this is how effectively foods as fuel can be grouped together in creating a lean body.

PREPARATION

We all lead busy lives, and yet we all operate under the same 24-hour clock. The difference is in how we choose to utilize our time. When trying to lose fat, for many it's less about getting to the gym and more about what to eat. What to prep and how are common issues. And yet with some simple tips, healthy food preparation is quite manageable and easy.

I generally do my food shopping for the week on Saturday mornings. Once I have all of my fuel in the kitchen, prep is nearly a cinch. I place my chicken breasts in a pan on the stove, sprinkling them with some spices to add flavor instead of calorie-dense oils. While the chicken is doing its thing, the microwave is cooking some yams/sweet potatoes. When they are finished, I microwave some green vegetables, such as asparagus. I scoop protein powder into shaker cups. My multivitamins and daily supplements go into a bag along with a fork and my raw almonds.

When everything is finished, I seal it all in airtight storage containers. When it's time to go to work, I just grab the sealed containers and drop them into a cooler with an ice pack. Buying pre-cooked items such as quinoa in bulk further eliminates prep time. My nutrition is like my training: linear, efficient and full of quality.

SAMPLE DAILY MENU

Here is a sample menu of an exact day of eating as I prepared for the photos in this book.

 8:00 AM:
- 2 whole eggs and 6 egg whites, scrambled and topped with salsa
- ready-made quinoa bowl
- black coffee with cinnamon and calorie-free sweetener

 11:00 AM:
- RTD (ready-to-drink) shake
- small handful raw almonds

 2:00 PM:
- 2 small chicken breasts seasoned with Cajun spice
- yam/sweet potato
- asparagus

 5:00 PM:
- RTD (ready-to-drink) shake
- small handful raw almonds

 8:00 PM:
- 2 pieces of cod seasoned with garlic powder
- ready-made brown rice bowl
- brussels sprouts

ON DELIVERY SERVICES

If you are low on time, choices for delicious, nutritious meals that are big on taste and fuel can be delivered right to your door. You can supplement your own cooking with services like The Life Chef (www.lalifechef.com) that cook up delicious, high-quality foods.

TRY IT AT HOME

You can also try these recipes for yourself. They are easy, and take little time to prepare. (*Recipes provided by The Life Chef at www.lalifechef.com*).

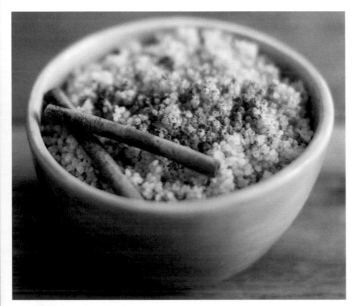

Cinnamon Quinoa Hot Cereal / *280 calories, 9g fat, 40g carbs, 8g protein*

CINNAMON QUINOA HOT CEREAL

Serves 1–2

Ingredients

1 cup (200g) cooked quinoa

½ tablespoon coconut oil

½ –1 cup (120–240ml) unsweetened coconut milk

(add milk to desired consistency)

1–2 teaspoons cinnamon

½ teaspoon vanilla extract

- Mix all ingredients in pan and heat until hot. Stir occasionally to mix ingredients.

- Pour into bowl, add preferred nuts or berries and enjoy.

THREE-BEAN SALAD

Serves 2

Ingredients

½ cup (100g) kidney beans

½ cup (100g) white beans

½ cup (100g) garbanzo beans/chickpeas

2 garlic cloves, chopped

⅛ cup (25g) red onion, finely chopped

2 tablespoons chopped green onion

2 tablespoons chopped parsley

2 tablespoons apple cider vinegar

2 tablespoons olive oil

½ teaspoon salt

black pepper to taste

- Combine the beans and chopped items in mixing bowl.

- In small bowl, mix olive oil, vinegar, salt and pepper.

- Add dressing to mix and toss.

For best results chill 2–3 hours to let beans marinate.

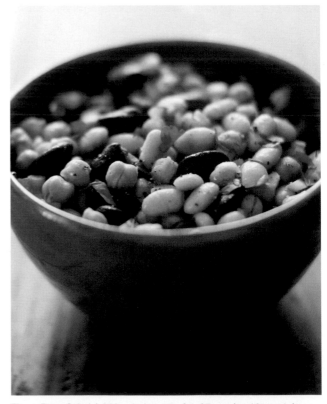

Three-Bean Salad / *283 calories, 15g fat, 27g carbs, 10g protein*

DIJON SALMON

Serves 4

Ingredients

1½ pounds (700g) salmon
2 tablespoons fresh parsley, finely chopped
2–3 small cloves of garlic, pressed
1½ teaspoons Dijon mustard
½ teaspoon salt
⅛ teaspoon freshly ground black pepper
⅛ cup (30ml) olive oil
2 tablespoons fresh lemon juice
lemon slices

- Preheat oven to 450°F/230°C and line a rimmed baking dish with aluminium foil.

- In a small bowl, combine the parsley, garlic, Dijon mustard, salt, pepper, olive oil and lemon juice. Mix well.

- Cut salmon into even portions and lay them onto your lined baking dish skin side down.

- Generously brush all sides of your salmon with the sauce and top with fresh lemon slices.

- Bake at 450°F/230°C for 10–12 minutes.

- Remove lemon slices and serve with Sautéed Lemon Kale (see page 43) and quinoa garnished with avocado.

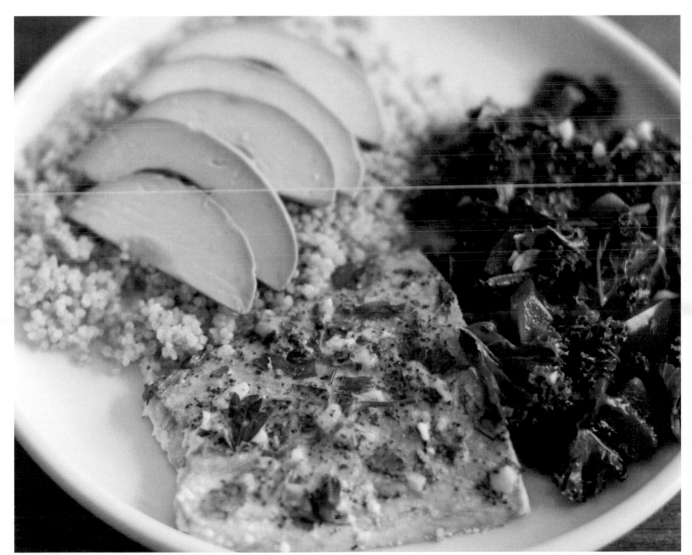

Dijon Salmon / *496 calories 25g fat, 4g carbs, 37g protein*

LEMON PEPPER AND THYME CHICKEN

Serves 4

Ingredients

1½ tablespoons lemon juice
¼ teaspoon dried thyme or 1 tablespoon fresh thyme
½ teaspoon dried red pepper flakes
1 clove garlic, minced
¼ cup (50g) olive oil
¼ teaspoon salt
¼ teaspoon fresh-ground black pepper
4 chicken breasts (1½–2 pounds)

- Preheat grill or heat the broiler.
- In a shallow dish, combine the lemon juice with the thyme, red pepper flakes, garlic, oil, salt and black pepper. Coat the chicken with the mixture.
- Grill the chicken breasts over moderately high heat or broil them for 8–12 minutes.
- Remove from heat, and serve with rice and beans or a side dish of your choice.

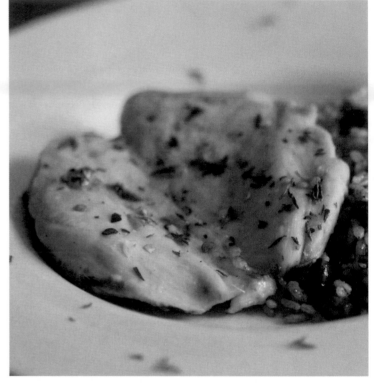

Lemon Pepper and Thyme Chicken / *330 calories, 16g fat, 5g carbs, 39g protein*

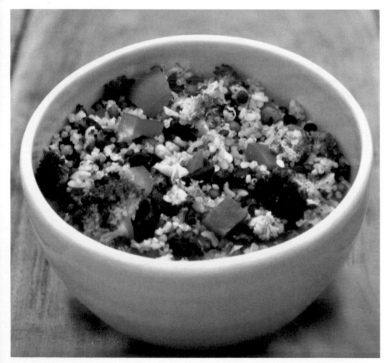

Vegan Protein and Veggie Bowl / *258 calories, 14g fat, 26g carbs, 7g protein*

VEGAN PROTEIN AND VEGGIE BOWL

Serves 2

Ingredients

¼ cup (50g) cooked brown rice
¼ cup (50g) cooked quinoa
¼ cup (50g) cooked lentils
¼ cup (50g) black beans
3 garlic cloves
¼ cup (50g) chopped yellow onion
¼ cup (50g) chopped red bell pepper
1 cup chopped broccoli
2 tablespoons olive oil
½ teaspoon cayenne pepper
salt and pepper to taste

- Sauté the garlic, onion, peppers and broccoli in a pan.
- Add rest of ingredients and mix thoroughly in pan until beans are coated and warmed.

CURRIED CAULIFLOWER

Serves 2

Ingredients

4 cups (800g) chopped
cauliflower
1 tablespoon olive or
coconut oil
2 teaspoons curry powder
salt and black pepper
to taste

- Preheat oven to 425°F/220°C.

- Combine all ingredients in
  mixing bowl and toss until all
  ingredients are mixed well.

- Roast covered in an oven-
  safe dish for 25–40 minutes,
  depending on desired firmness
  of cauliflower (the longer you
  roast the softer it becomes).

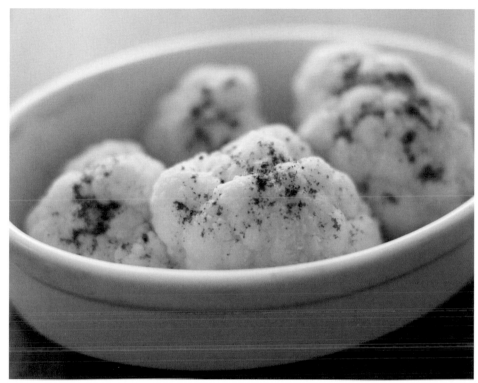

Curried Cauliflower / *120 calories, 7g fat, 10g carbs, 4g protein*

LENTIL SCRAMBLE

Serves 1

Ingredients

½ cup (100g) cooked lentils
2 whole eggs or 4 egg whites
2 garlic cloves
⅛ cup (25g) chopped red onion
⅛ cup (25g) red bell pepper
1 small Roma/plum tomato
½ cup (50g) chopped spinach
½ teaspoon turmeric
½ avocado

- Spray pan with coconut or olive oil spray
  and sauté the garlic, onions, peppers,
  tomato and spinach.

- Add turmeric and lentil, and stir well.

- Add eggs and scramble.

- Top with sliced avocado.

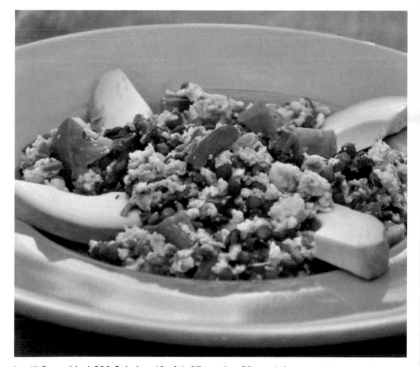

Lentil Scramble / *290 Calories, 10g fat, 27g carbs, 23g protein*

GARLIC AND BALSAMIC ROASTED BRUSSELS SPROUTS

Serves 2

Ingredients

Extra virgin olive oil
3 cloves chopped garlic
2 cups (400g) halved brussels sprouts
⅛ cup balsamic vinegar
salt and pepper to taste

- Preheat oven to 425°F/220°C.
- In a large mixing bowl, combine all ingredients and toss a few times.
- Place mixed ingredients into oven-safe dish, and roast covered for 15 minutes.
- Uncover and stir ingredients.
- Place back in oven and continue to roast uncovered for another 20–30 minutes, depending on the size of the brussels sprouts.

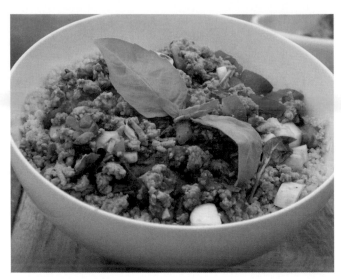

Turkey and Quinoa Bowl / *478 calories, 22.5g fat, 31g carbs, 35g protein*

TURKEY AND QUINOA BOWL

Serves 4–5

Ingredients

1½ pounds (700g) ground turkey meat
1½ cups (300g) cooked quinoa
4 Roma/plum tomatoes, chopped
½ bell pepper
⅛ cup (25g) fresh basil, chopped
4 cloves garlic
½ red or sweet onion
⅛ cup (25g) green onion/spring onion
2 tablespoons olive oil
½ cup (100g) chopped zucchini/courgette
½ cup (100g) chopped yellow squash
1 cup (200g) chopped spinach

- In a large saucepan over medium heat, lightly sauté the garlic and onions.
- Add the turkey meat and begin to brown.
- Add tomatoes, zucchini/courgette, squash, spinach, basil and bell pepper.
- Continue to cook covered, stirring occasionally until turkey is cooked through, about 6–8 minutes.
- Place cooked quinoa in bowl and pour ingredients from pan over it.
- Top with your favorite pasta sauce and garnish with fresh basil leaves.

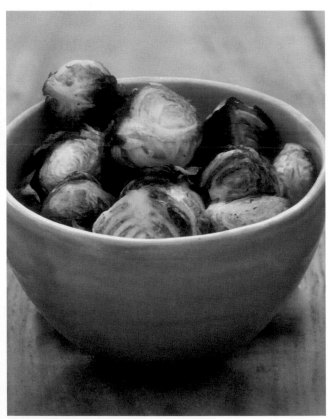

Garlic and Balsamic Roasted Brussels Sprouts /
150 calories, 9g fat, 12g carbs, 3g protein

SAUTÉED LEMON KALE
Serves 2

Ingredients
4 cups (200g) chopped kale
2 cloves of garlic
½ chopped red bell pepper
¼ cup sweet onion, chopped
juice from ½ lemon
1 tablespoon coconut or olive oil
sea salt to taste

- Heat pan with oil on medium heat.
- Add the garlic, bell peppers and onion and sauté for about 1 minute.
- Add kale and lemon juice.
- Cover with lid and occasionally. Stir and fold ingredients.
- Cook for 3–4 minutes, until the kale begins to turn bright green.
- Add salt to taste.

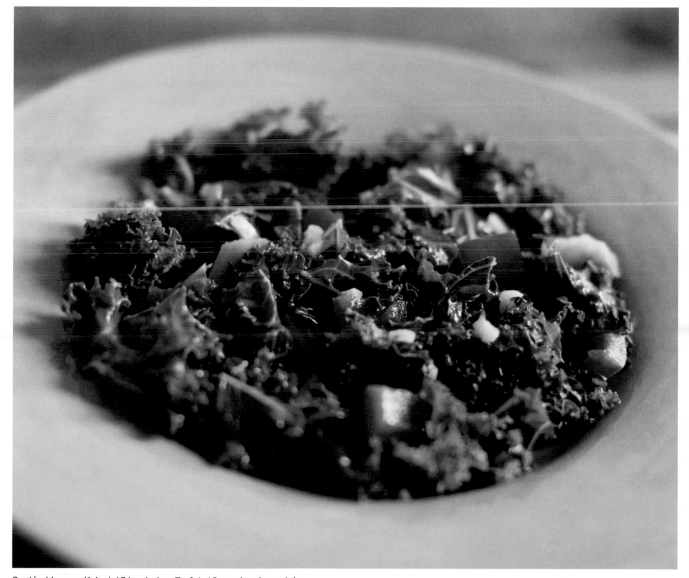

Sautéed Lemon Kale / *151 calories, 7g fat, 18g carbs, 4g protein*

ON EATING OUT

For many of us, it is easy to eat cleanly at home. But once in a restaurant, the rules of the game are often thrown out. Unless you're using your dining out as a cheat meal (more on this later), you absolutely can stick to your program in nearly every possible situation, while you enjoy being social and feeling satiated. And all without the guilt.

STEAK RESTAURANTS

Order a less-marbled cut of beef and opt for top round or flank steak. Or go grilled with chicken or seafood. Add an unadorned baked potato (make sure they did not pre-spray with butter) and a steamed vegetable.

CHINESE

Order your favorite dish steamed and ask for brown rice, which many of these establishments now serve. Have sauce sparingly on the side.

FAST FOOD

Order a grilled chicken salad without cheese or heavy dressing or a grilled chicken breast with lettuce and tomato or a plain hamburger.

SUB PLACE

Order turkey or chicken breast on whole wheat with lettuce, tomato, black olives (good source of fat), peppers and mustard. Avoid the tuna fish—it's filled with fatty mayo!

ITALIAN

Chicken breast over whole-wheat pasta with dry salad. Avoid breads and heavy sauces.

ON SUPPLEMENTATION

Vitamins and supplements are a multibillion-dollar business. My own personal take is that supplements are just that: supplemental. Your nutrition should cover most, if not all of the bases. But it never hurts to have extra assurances as well as making sure you're taking in all the essentials, especially while on your peaking journey.

For our purposes here, I will share with you what I personally take and why, rather than blindly recommending any items to my readers. I feel good about the following choices, and believe that more is not better—otherwise it ends up as expensive urine—and that a logical approach should be taken to supplementation. If you are unsure where to start, having your doctor run a vitamin-deficiency test may not be a bad idea.

Multivitamins

For those who regularly workout, one pill claiming to contain all one needs is not going to cut it. A packet with a grouping of different vitamins and minerals is the ticket.

Fish oil

For skin, hair, heart. Good fats do a body good.

Glucosamine/chondroitin

I do believe these supplements help with the lubrication of my joints and improve their elasticity while also helping to reinforce them for the wear and tear that years of progressive resistance training can result in.

Protein powder

This is an inexpensive way to get protein efficiently. I prefer casein (slow digesting) as opposed to whey (quick digesting). And ladies, I do count this extra protein as a meal (in addition to my almonds), and it will not turn you into an overnight Hercules.

Pre-workout powder

This is definitely not for those with pre-existing heart conditions or hypertension. I use this family of supplements in combination with real food to help power me through my workouts. Let's be honest here, and admit that sometimes it's very difficult to hit a home run. Pre-workout powders, along with loud music, nearly always ensure that I at least get up to the plate for a good swing.

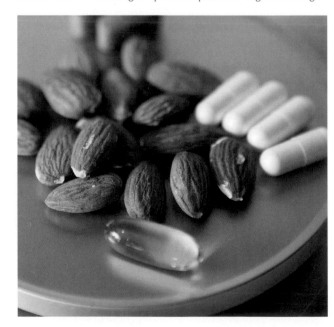

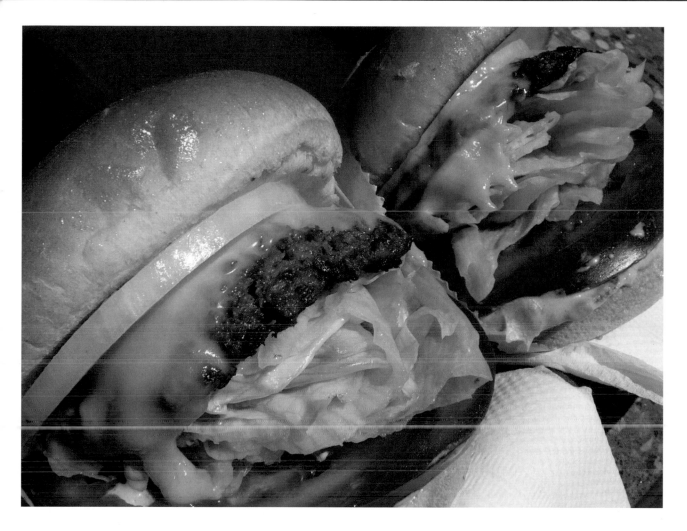

THE CHEAT MEAL

As your body adapts to the journey toward peak condition, it can sometimes take weeks for you to see even subtle changes. And once progress begins, there will of course be weeks in which little to no change occurs. Keep on course. Progressive change is imminent.

I do feel it necessary, both physically and mentally, to loosen the dietary belt at least once per week. Anticipating a treat will help alleviate the day-in-day-out mental strain of your program. You will know that you have something fabulously sinful coming your way weekly, an indulgence that you have indeed earned.

To me the cheat meal is like a holy experience, one in which I would almost always prefer to enjoy alone. It's like that game-show segment in which a contestant, sealed in a confined space, has mere seconds to grab as much loose cash as possible while money is blown in and rains down.

I generally give myself one hour to siphon down all the delectable goodies I can hold.

Psychologically, the best part of the cheat meal is when you know that an eating extravaganza is imminent. It is the same high that a gambler experiences as the dice is in motion. That anticipation feels almost as sinful and delicious as the very first bite. While some are able to indulge in one chip or one cookie, for others scarfing an entire bag of chips or cookies is merely a prelude to the main act. To this I say, eat clean most of the time, but when you're going to cheat, do it as if it's your last supper. Fully satiate your cravings, getting the urge to splurge out of your system until the next allotted cheat meal.

What I am asking of you is that once a week, enjoy one meal—and one meal only—of whatever you desire. This good monkey wrench, if you will, actually speeds up your metabolism. So, indulge, and then get right back on track.

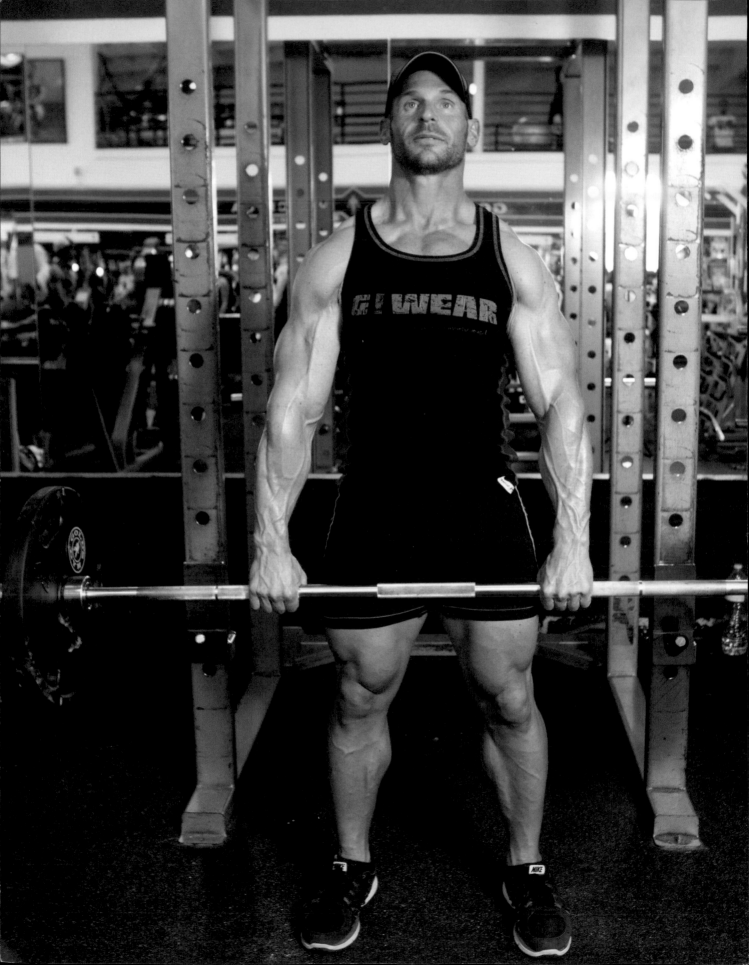

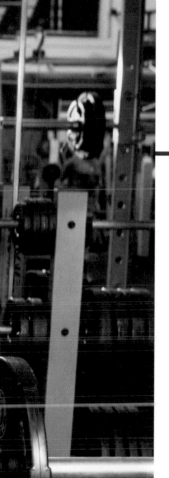

CHAPTER 5

GYM WORKOUTS

The following exercises have been selected and grouped for their effectiveness. The included movements are representative of the actual functions of your muscles, how they work best at enhancing your genetic shape, efficiently stimulating temporary muscular failure, and keeping you lean. They are also my personal favorites; over the years, I, along with countless clients, have seen great success with them.

Aside from the safe completion of each workout, the most important points to consider while performing these exercises are that you are firing from the correct muscles, utilizing a full range of motion and breathing throughout each repetition. The scope of your workouts, although not overtly expansive, is thorough in readying you for your best. Additionally, these workouts are unisex in design. Women now know that the days of ineffectively lifting tiny little weights are long past, and men know to check their egos at the door. We all share the same muscles, so you can feel good and confident about the overall structure of your program.

A THOROUGH WORKOUT

The workouts featured in this chapter are more thorough in scope than those in chapter 6, and they will offer you the most bang for your buck when you have access to a gym. Each subsequent set of a given exercise should have increasing resistance and decreasing repetitions for the prescribed number of sets.

MACHINES VERSUS FREE WEIGHTS

In the eternal debate of machines versus free weights, I am often asked the question of which is better. Although some machines, such as the Lat Pulldown and Leg Press, are highly effective and indispensable pieces of equipment, they require less coordination than free weights and also follow a predetermined range of motion. As such, they are quite isolating. In addition, machines tend to be faster paced than free weights—simply placing a pin in a weight stack can change the resistance more efficiently than changing plates on a barbell.

Free weights, on the other hand, follow a vast range of angles and motions, as well as work ancillary or helper muscles along with the primary movers that machines exclude. They are much more versatile than machines: consider the near limitless exercise combinations you can perform with dumbbells. I also believe that using free weights more often than machines results in better muscle control and a higher-quality look to the physique, as well as faster results. For these reasons, the bulk of your routine is composed of basic, free-weight exercises to provide you with not only an effective workout but also a complete look to your physique.

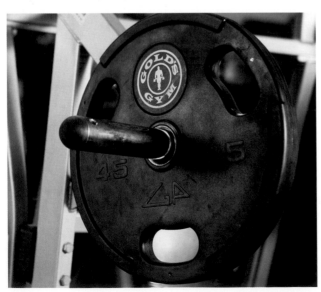

SLOW AND STEADY

The word *speed* should be eliminated from your fitness vocabulary. Although efficiency and expediency are important parts of your workout, your goal is to train each specific muscle group only once a week, 12 times per muscle group for the duration of this program. You must make each and every workout count—make sure that you are mentally present and willing to put the tension on that particular day's muscles without recruiting other muscles, which can result in injury. In the build-up to each set, always take a moment to ensure a proper set-up. Just as a speaker centers him- or herself in the middle of a room prior to speaking, set your body properly prior to lifting. This entire program calls for a realistic commitment from you. Give that commitment, and it will deliver realistic and noticeable results.

Will you have heavily defined abdominals, broad shoulders and a tapering waist at the conclusion of this program? That depends on your starting point, genetics and how much you're willing to put into it. Do I guarantee that you will have noticeable changes to even the untrained eye? If you stay committed to this program and run its course, absolutely.

PERIPHERALS

Just as every sport or vocation has its tools to help get the job done, there exists an arsenal of available items to help support your exercise endeavors. Clothing can act as inspiration: while you're in the sporting goods shop, take the time to try on workout outfits that will flatter your future physique. Although not required, certain equipment acts as not only a line of defense (weight belt), but will also ensure that your muscles give out before your grip does (straps). Here are a few recruits that have helped me over the years.

Belt

The weight-lifting belt is so effective, we see its usage outside of the gym. It's present on construction sites, worn by workers doing the heavy lifting, and in supermarkets, worn by parents carrying their babies. The belt offers support to the lumbar region and is particularly useful for overhead movements and squats. A word of caution: never wear a belt during the Leg Press.

Straps

Wrist straps ensure that your back muscles give out before the weak links, your grip and forearms, do. This will allow you to perform extra repetitions—and extra repetitions means extra muscular stimulation.

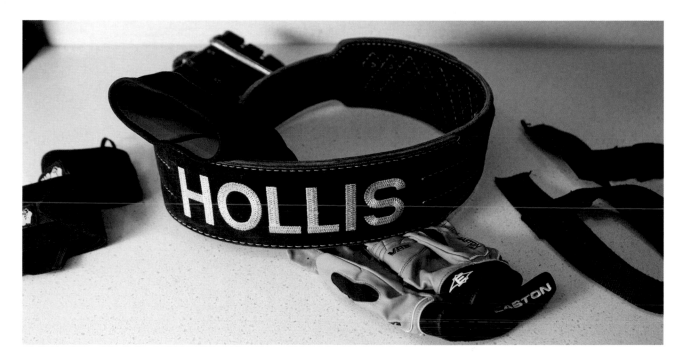

Gloves

Gloves can provide padded protection when gripping the cold steel and keep calluses away.

Elbow sleeve

Although a later addition to my arsenal, a slip-on elbow sleeve, with its supportive compression over sore elbows and triceps, has made continual pressing movements possible.

ACTION BY PHASE

There are three phases to your program, each lasting four weeks. Each new phase adds subtle changes in exercise duration and intensity, which builds slowly over time so that you not only adapt, but also advance. Keep track of the resistance you employ, which should increase over time. Remember that lifting heavier weights actually burns more calories than lighter loads.

What follows below are each of the three training phases outlined in their entirety for your complete program and its advancements. Each exercise is listed in its order of appearance for each of the four-week training blocks. Each and every exercise is further broken down into proper performance, suggested sets and repetition ranges. Phase 1 is based largely on the super-setting principal (when practical). In a superset, you perform one exercise back to back with another for all of the suggested sets and repetitions (followed by a brief rest in between)

before moving onto the next pair of exercises. Phases 2 and 3 follow a more traditional approach, utilizing straight sets. Here you perform a set, rest, and then perform the next working set of the same exercise until all sets are completed. You then advance to the next exercise. All you have to supply is the resistance and sweat.

THE HUMAN JENGA

It is human nature to want to do everything at once. As you've learned by now, getting into shape is about doing precisely what needs to be done on a daily basis over time to ensure not only the best results, but also long-term results. It is also about skilled manipulation in what I call "The Jenga Equation," in which one or two pieces are slowly changed over time. This way the foundation remains sturdy or, in our case here, progressive. But if too many pieces are manipulated at once, the house topples.

The last week before your event will never make a huge difference if you haven't done your homework prior to the big dance. But having followed this program, you can expect to make a subtle enhancement during the last week. Assuming your event is on a Saturday, final preparation starts on the prior Wednesday. Simply drop all condiments and seasonings from your nutritional intake, drink extra spring water to flush your system of sodium and consume extra asparagus, which is a natural diuretic, and coast into your event feeling and looking great.

THE WORKOUTS

The following lists outline the three phases of your Peak Physique gym workout program, detailing which exercises to perform and on which day.

Each day of the week will be either a rest day or a workout day. For each workout day, the target area is listed, along with the recommended cardio duration.

Next, you will find a list of exercises. Each exercise has corresponding numbers next to it indicating the total number of sets and repetitions you should perform. For example, "Seated Dumbbell Press 3X 8–12" translates to "three sets of 8 to 12 repetitions."

When you see "superset" listed, as in "Cable Flye *superset* with Dumbbell Pullover 2X 8–15," this translates to "both exercises performed back to back for two sets of 8 to 15 repetitions of both exercises."

PHASE 1
WEEKS 1–4
BEGINNER TRAINING PROTOCOL

MONDAY
Target: Chest/Back/Abdominals
Cardio: 30 minutes
Exercises:
- Incline Barbell Press *superset* with Front Pulldown 3X 8–12
- Hammer Strength Flat Press *superset* with Dumbbell Row 3X 8–12
- Cable Flye *superset* with Dumbbell Pullover 2X 8–15
- Pec Deck *superset* with Reverse Hyperextension 2X 12–15
- Crunch *superset* with Reverse Crunch 2X 20–25

TUESDAY: REST

WEDNESDAY
Target: Legs
Cardio: 30 minutes
Exercises:
- Smith Machine Squat 3X 12–15
- Alternate Reverse Lunge 2X 12–15
- Leg Extension 2X 12–15
- Lying Leg Curl 3X 1–12
- Seated Leg Curl 2X 12–15
- Standing Calf Raise 3X 12–15

THURSDAY: REST

FRIDAY
Target: Shoulders/Arms/Abdominals
Cardio: 30 minutes
Exercises:
- Seated Dumbbell Press 3X 8–12
- Standing Lateral Raise 2X 10–12
- Reverse Flye 2X 10–12
- Upright Row 2X 10–12
- Standing Alternate Dumbbell Curl *superset* with Lying Triceps Extension 2X 10–12
- Rope Hammer Curl *superset* with Overhead Dumbbell Extensions 2X 10–12
- Preacher Curl *superset* Triceps Pushdown 2X 10–15
- Down-Up *superset* with Seated Russian Twist 2X 15–20

SATURDAY: REST

SUNDAY: REST

PHASE 2
WEEKS 5-8
INTERMEDIATE TRAINING PROTOCOL

MONDAY
Target: Chest/Triceps/Abdominals
Cardio: 30 minutes
Exercises:
- Incline Barbell Press 3X 8–12
- Hammer Strength Flat Press 3X 8–12
- Cable Flye 2X 12–15
- Pec Deck 2X 12–15
- Cable Crossover 2X 12–15
- Lying Triceps Extension 2X 10–12
- Overhead Dumbbell Extension 2X 10–12
- Triceps Pushdown 2X 12–15
- Crunch *superset* Reverse Crunch 2X 20–25

TUESDAY
Target: Back
Cardio: 30 minutes
Exercises:
- Front Pull-Down 3X 8–12
- Dumbbell Row 3X 8–12
- T-Bar Row 2X 8–12
- Dumbbell Pullover 2X 8–12
- Reverse Hyperextension 2X 12–15

WEDNESDAY: REST

THURSDAY

Target: Legs/Abdominals

Cardio: 30 minutes

Exercises:

- Hack Squat 3X 12–15
- Leg Press 3X 12–15
- Alternate Reverse Lunge 2X 12–15
- Leg Extension 2X 12–15
- Lying Leg Curl 3X 10–12
- Seated Leg Curl 2X 12–15
- One-Legged Curl 2X 12–15
- Standing Calf Raise 3X 12–15
- Crunch *superset* with Down-Ups 2X 15–25

FRIDAY

Target: Shoulders/Biceps/Abdominals

Cardio: 30 minutes

Exercises:

- Seated Dumbbell Press 3X 8–12
- Front Barbell Raise 2X 10–12
- Standing Lateral Raise 2X 10–12
- Reverse Flye 2X 10–12
- Upright Row 2X 10–12
- Standing Alternate Dumbbell Curl 2X 10–12
- Rope Hammer Curl 2X 10–12
- Preacher Curl 2X 10–12
- Reverse Crunch *superset* with Seated Russian Twist 2X 20

SATURDAY: REST

SUNDAY: REST

PHASE 3
WEEKS 9–12
ADVANCED TRAINING PROTOCOL

MONDAY

Target: Chest/Triceps/Abdominals

Cardio: 40 minutes

Exercises:

- Incline Barbell Press 3X 8–12
- Hammer Strength Flat Press 3X 8–12
- Cable Flye 2X 12–15
- Pec Deck 2X 12–15
- Cable Crossover 2X 12–15
- Lying Triceps Extension 2X 10–12
- Overhead Dumbbell Extension 2X 10–12
- Triceps Pushdown 2X 12–15
- Dumbbell Kickback 2X 12–15
- Crunch *superset* Reverse Crunch 2X 20–25

TUESDAY

Target: Back

Cardio: 40 minutes

Exercises:

- Pull-Up 2X 8–10
- Barbell Row 2X 8–12
- T-Bar Row 2X 8–12
- Dumbbell Pullover 2X 8–12
- Reverse Hyperextension 2X 12–15
- Deadlift 2X 8–10

WEDNESDAY: REST

THURSDAY

Target: Legs/Abdominals

Cardio: 40 minutes

Exercises:

- Smith Machine Squats (Feet shoulder-width) 2X 12–15
- Hack Squat (Feet close) 2X 12–15
- Leg Press 3X 12–15
- Alternate Reverse Lunge 2X 12–15
- Leg Extension 2X 12–15
- Lying Leg Curl 3X 10–12
- Seated Leg Curl 2X 12–15
- One-Legged Curl 2X 12–15
- Standing Calf Raise 3X 12–15
- Crunch superset with Down-Up 2X 15–25

FRIDAY

Target: Shoulders/Biceps/Abdominals

Cardio: 40 minutes

Exercises:

- Seated Dumbbell Press 3X 8–12
- Front Barbell Raise 2X 10–12
- Standing Lateral Raise 2X 10–12
- Reverse Flye 2X 10–12
- Upright Row 2X 10–12
- Standing Alternate Dumbbell Curl 2X 10–12
- Rope Hammer Curl 2X 10–12
- Preacher Curl 2X 10–12
- One-Arm Cable Curl 2X 12–15
- Reverse Crunch superset with Seated Russian Twists 2X 20

SATURDAY

Cardio: 40 minutes

SUNDAY: REST

INCLINE BARBELL PRESS

PROGRESSION

1 Begin lying back on an incline bench with your feet planted on the ground and a shoulder-width grip on a barbell.

2 Start by lowering the barbell to your upper chest.

3 Push back up to full extension for 8 to 12 repetitions.

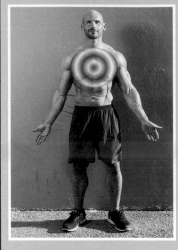

**MUSCLE ACTION:
PRIMARY ACTIVATION**
- pectoralis major

ANCILLARY ACTIVATION
- deltoideus anterior
- triceps brachii
- rectus abdominis
- erector spinae
- transversus abdominis

PROPER FORM
- A controlled lowering
- Bringing the barbell to your upper chest
- Your feet on the ground

BEGINNER MODIFICATION
- Arching your back
- Bouncing the bar off your chest
- Excessive speed

BEGINNER MODIFICATION
- A wider grip will decrease the range of motion.

ADVANCED MODIFICATION
- A closer grip will increase the range of motion.

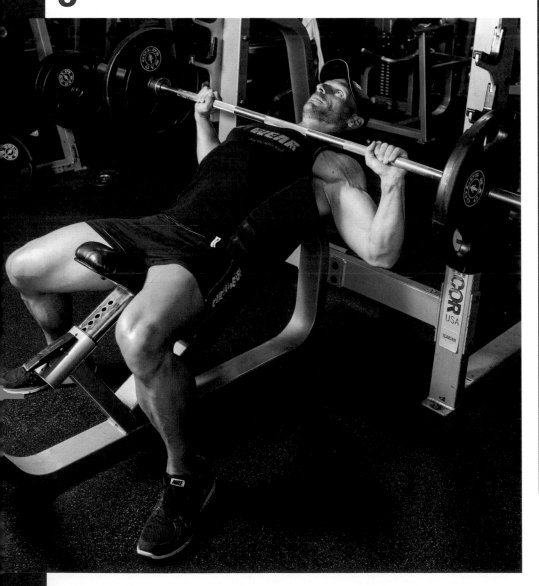

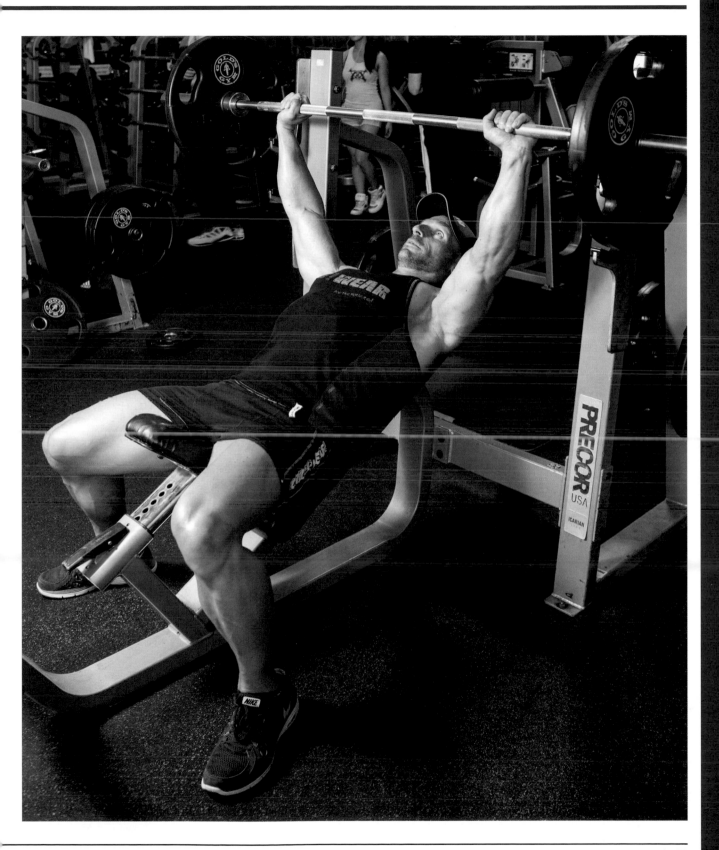

HAMMER STRENGTH FLAT PRESS

PROGRESSION

1 Begin seated in a Hammer Strength Machine with your feet planted on the ground and your hands on the grips with your knuckles in line with your nipple line.

2 Start by pushing the grips away from you for a full extension until your chest is in the fully contracted position.

3 Return to the starting position for 8 to 12 repetitions.

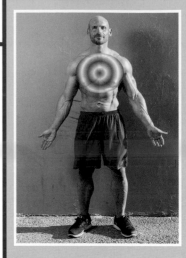

MUSCLE ACTION: PRIMARY ACTIVATION
- pectoralis major

ANCILLARY ACTIVATION
- deltoideus anterior
- triceps brachii
- rectus abdominis
- erector spinae
- transversus abdominis

PROPER FORM
- A full extension
- A controlled lowering
- Your knuckles in line with your nipple line

AVOID
- Bouncy or incomplete repetitions
- A fast or sloppy return to the starting position
- Not keeping your lower back braced

BEGINNER MODIFICATION
- A wider grip will decrease the range of motion.

ADVANCED MODIFICATION
- A closer grip will increase the range of motion.

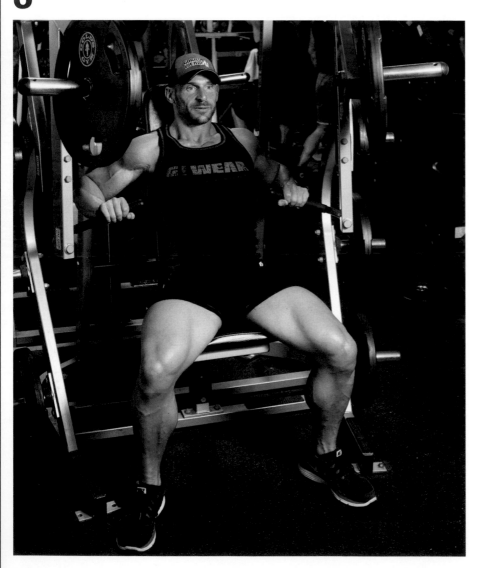

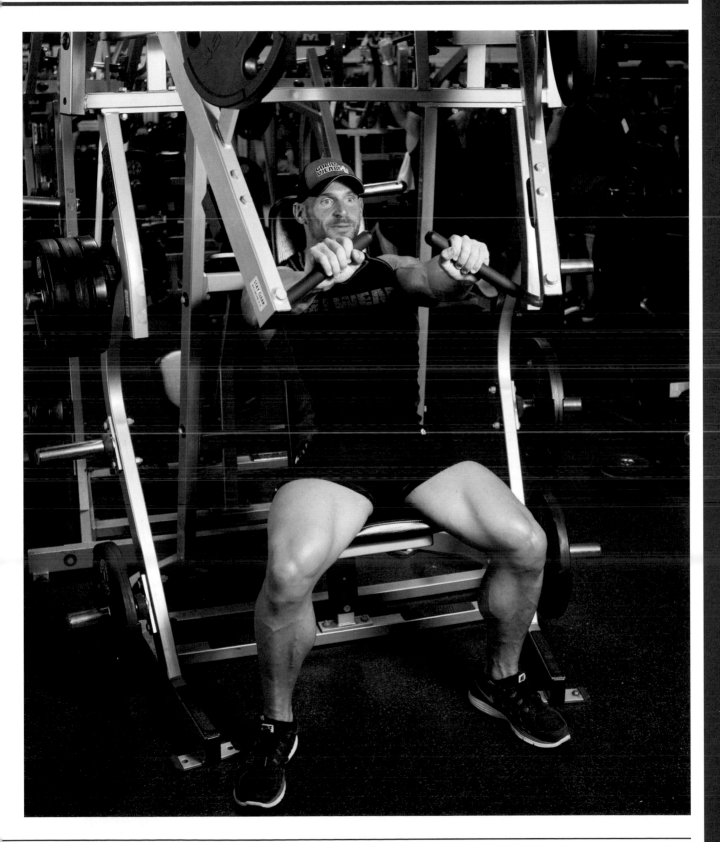

CABLE FLYE

PROGRESSION

1 Begin on your back on a flat bench placed in the middle of a cable stack with your feet planted on the ground, and grip the handles.

2 With the handles directly over your chest pushed to full extension, bend your arms as you move the handles away from your body in an arc.

3 In a hug-like motion, return the handles to the starting position, lengthening your arms the closer you get to center for 12 to 15 repetitions.

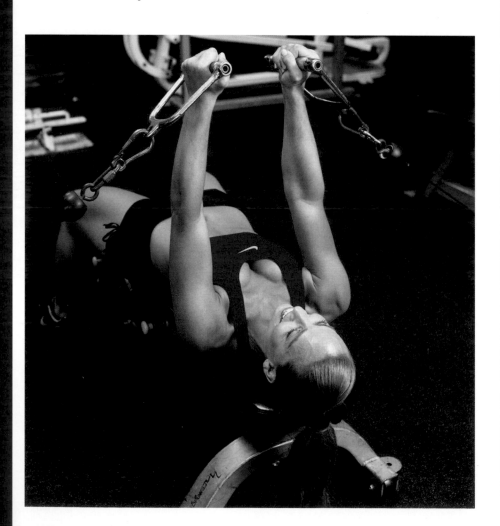

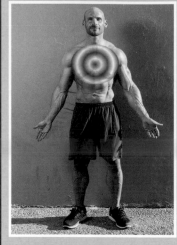

**MUSCLE ACTION:
PRIMARY ACTIVATION**
- pectoralis major

ANCILLARY ACTIVATION
- deltoideus anterior
- triceps brachii
- rectus abdominis
- erector spinae
- transversus abdominis

PROPER FORM
- A controlled lowering of the cables
- Squeezing your pecs together at the top of the movement
- Keeping your arms slightly bent during the outward phase of the exercise

AVOID
- Excessive speed or stretching
- Straightening your arms out to your sides
- Arching your back

BEGINNER MODIFICATION
- Try a lighter resistance.

ADVANCED MODIFICATION
- Try alternating one arm at a time.

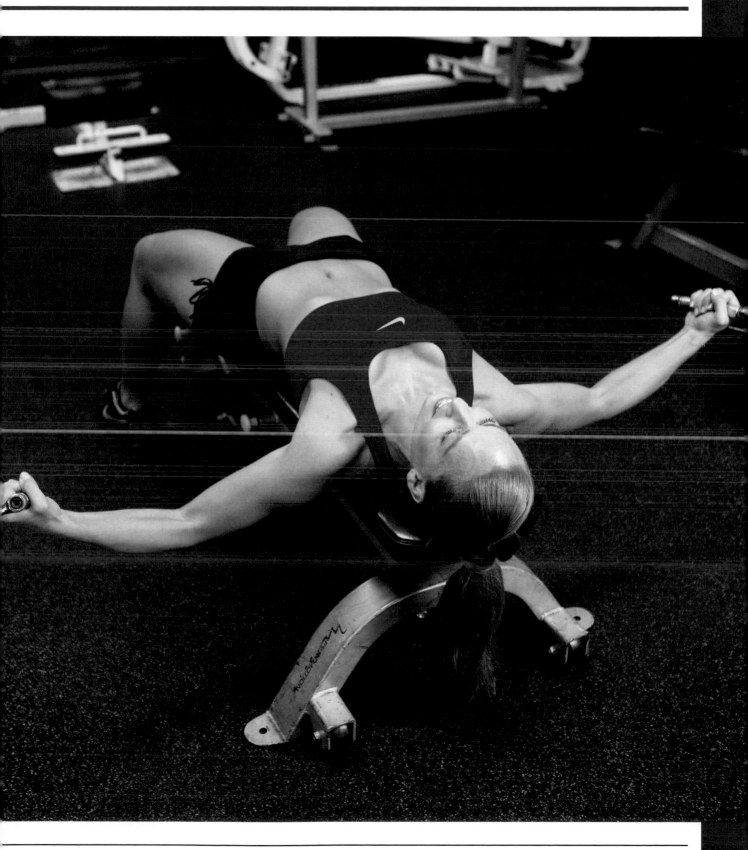

PEC DECK

PROGRESSION

1 Begin seated at a Pec Deck Machine with your lower back braced against the pad, both arms placed behind the arm slots, and your hands on the grips.

2 Bring both arms together while squeezing your chest, feeling the contraction as you repeat for 12 to 15 repetitions.

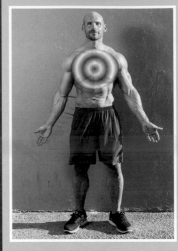

MUSCLE ACTION:
PRIMARY ACTIVATION
- pectoralis major

ANCILLARY ACTIVATION
- deltoideus anterior
- rectus abdominis

PROPER FORM
- A controlled opening stretch from the chest
- Keeping your torso stabilized
- Squeezing the chest in the contracted position of the exercise

AVOID
- Excessive speed
- Relying too much on your anterior deltoids
- Haphazardly slapping the weights together

BEGINNER MODIFICATION
- Try a lighter resistance.

ADVANCED MODIFICATION
- Try alternating one arm at a time.

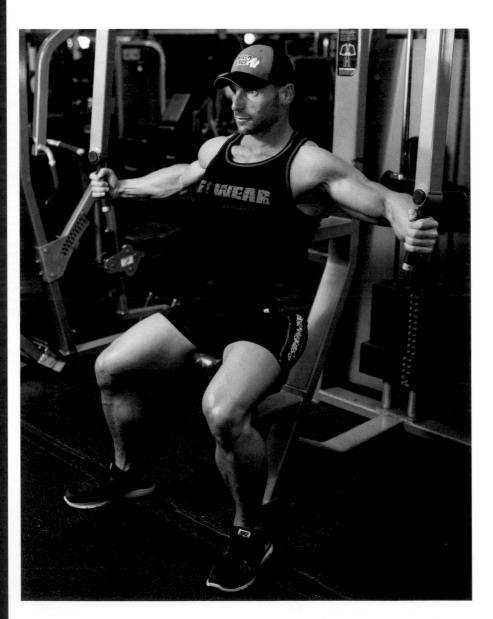

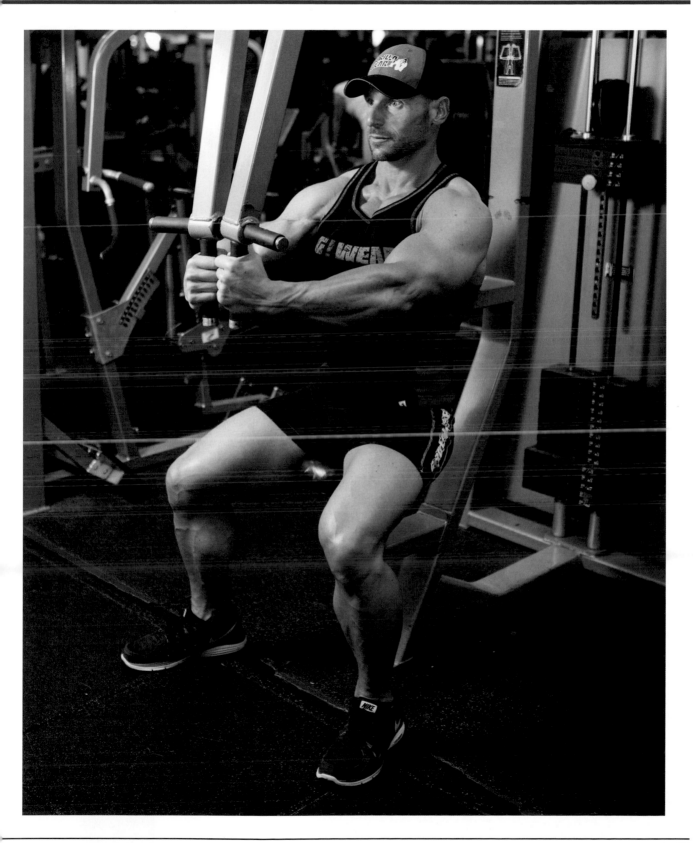

CABLE CROSSOVER

PROGRESSION

1 Begin standing in the middle of a pulley stack with the cables set at the high position, one handle in each hand, with one leg placed forward and the other backward.

2 Start by leaning forward and, while maintaining a flat back, draw your arms both down and across your chest until your knuckles are touching, feeling the muscles of your chest contract.

3 Contract your chest muscles, return your arms to the outstretched position in a controlled manner, and repeat for 12 to 15 repetitions.

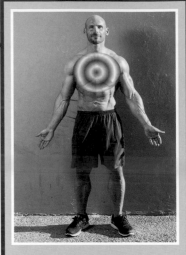

**MUSCLE ACTION:
PRIMARY ACTIVATION**
- pectoralis major

ANCILLARY ACTIVATION
- deltoideus anterior
- rectus abdominis
- rhomboideus

PROPER FORM
- A controlled lengthening of the arms
- Keeping your torso stabilized
- Maintaining a hugging motion throughout the exercise

AVOID
- Excessive speed
- The inclusion of too much anterior deltoids
- Leaning too far forward

BEGINNER MODIFICATION
- Try a lighter resistance.

ADVANCED MODIFICATION
- Try alternating one arm at a time.

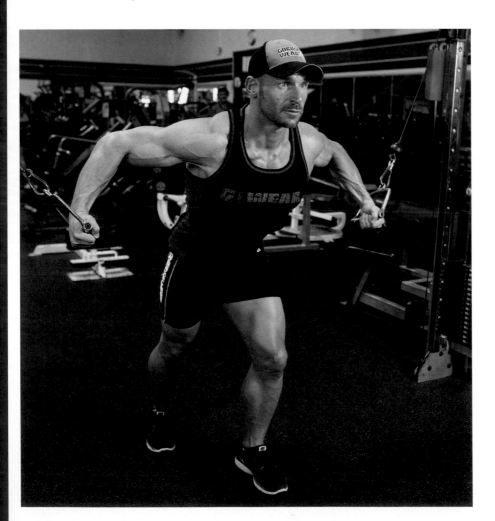

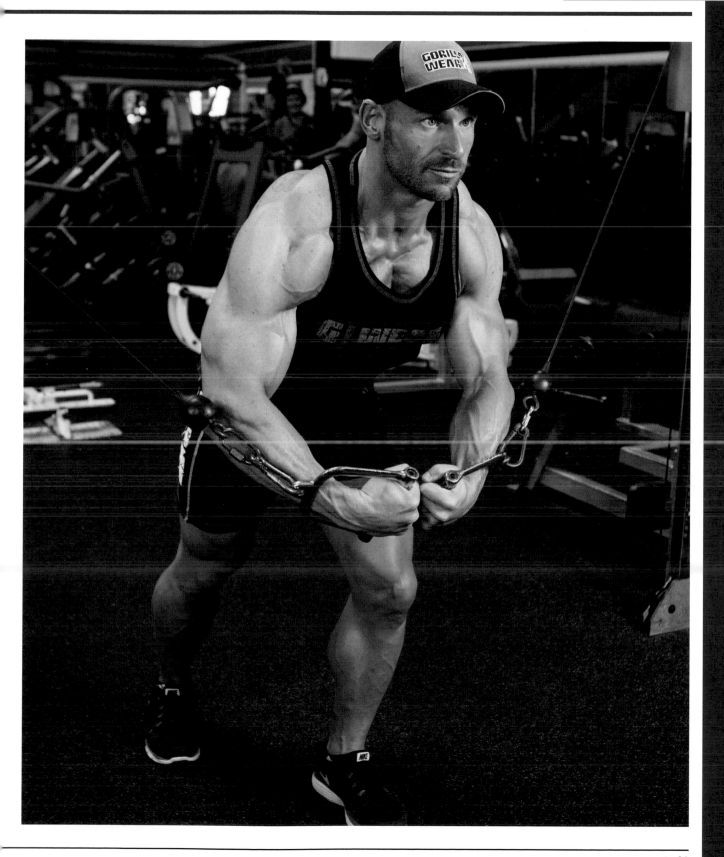

FRONT PULLDOWN

PROGRESSION

1 Begin seated at a Pulldown Machine while maintaining a shoulder-width, overhand grip on the bar attachment.

2 Pull the bar to the very top of your chest, while lowering your shoulders and then slowly extend the bar back up to full extension.

3 Complete the exercise for 8 to 12 repetitions.

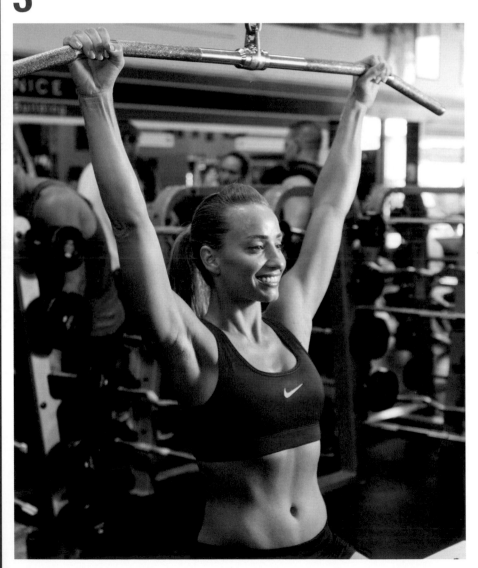

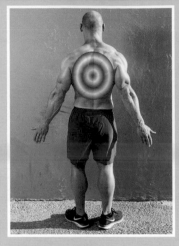

MUSCLE ACTION: PRIMARY ACTIVATION
- latissimus dorsi

ANCILLARY ACTIVATION
- trapezius
- biceps brachii
- rhomboideus
- forearm extensors
- forearm flexors

PROPER FORM
- A controlled and full range of motion
- Lowering your shoulders in the completed movement
- Keeping your back flat throughout the movement

AVOID
- Overarching your back
- Excessively swinging the weight
- Pulling behind the neck

BEGINNER MODIFICATION
- A wider grip will decrease the range of motion.

ADVANCED MODIFICATION
- A closer grip will increase the range of motion.

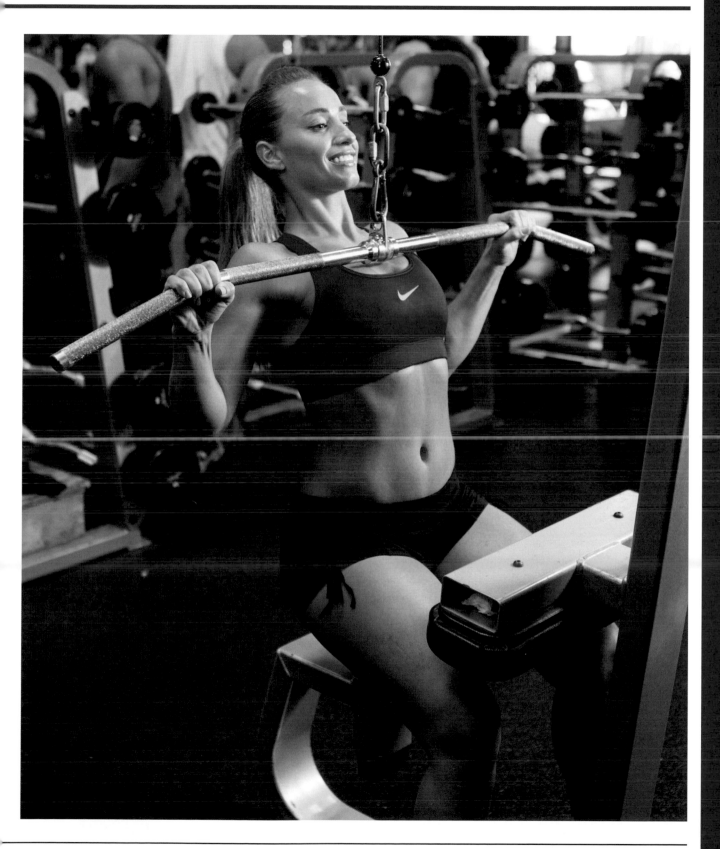

PULL-UP

PROGRESSION

1 Begin by standing in front of a pull-up bar and reach up or step on a stool to take an overhand, shoulder-width grip and hang below at arms' length.

2 Pull yourself up, bringing your chin as close to the bar as you can and then lower to arms' length. Repeat for 8 to 10 repetitions.

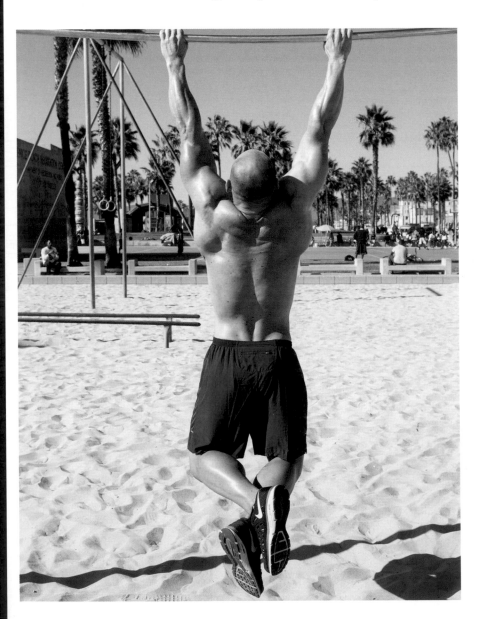

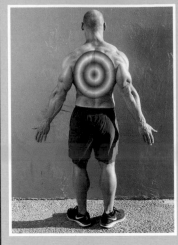

**MUSCLE ACTION:
PRIMARY ACTIVATION**
- latissimus dorsi

ANCILLARY ACTIVATION
- biceps brachii
- trapezius
- rhomboideus
- forearm extensors
- forearm flexors

PROPER FORM
- A controlled lowering or descent
- Pulling your chin to the bar
- Contracting each repetition at the top of the movement

AVOID
- Pulling behind your neck
- Excessive body swinging
- Using your arms instead of your back

BEGINNER MODIFICATION
- Have someone assist you at your legs.

ADVANCED MODIFICATION
- Try holding a light dumbbell between your lower legs.

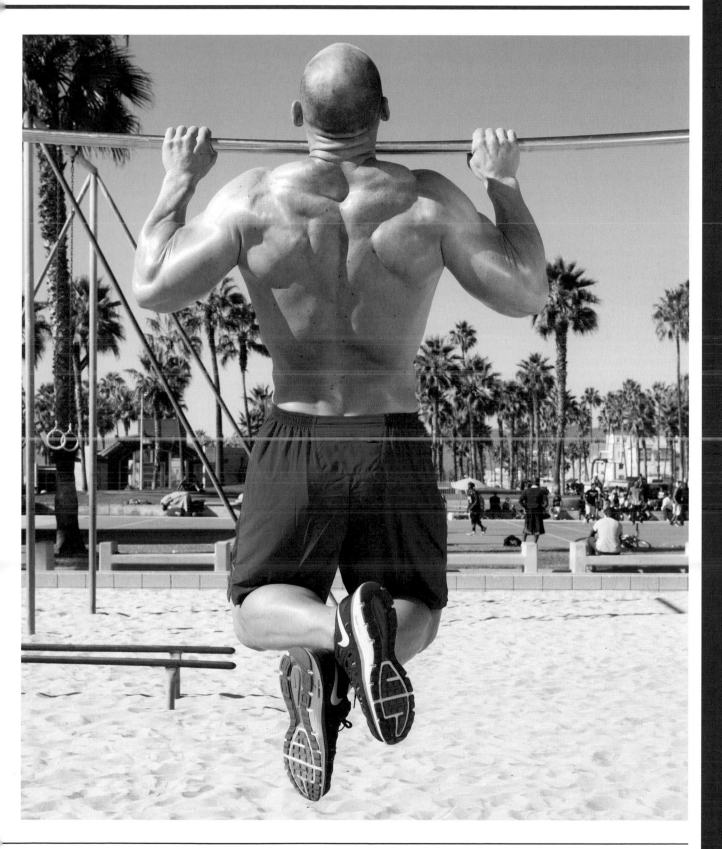

BARBELL ROW

PROGRESSION

1 Begin holding a barbell with an overhand grip, shoulder-width apart at arms' length.

2 Bend your knees slightly, with your rear pushed out, as you lean forward at the waist until your back is above parallel to the ground.

3 Start by bringing your arms back as you pull the bar into your midriff, contracting the lats hard.

4 Lower the barbell back down to full extension and then repeat the exercise for 8 to 12 full length repetitions.

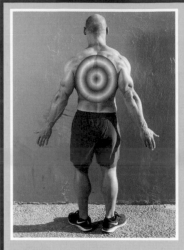

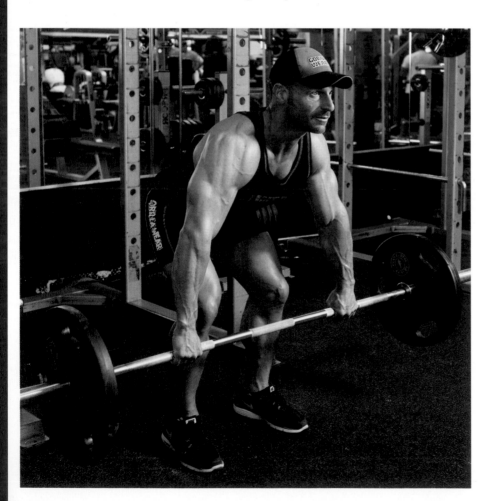

**MUSCLE ACTION:
PRIMARY ACTIVATION**
- upper back
- outer back

ANCILLARY ACTIVATION
- biceps brachii
- deltoideus posterior
- rhomboideus
- forearm extensors
- forearm flexors

PROPER FORM
- Maintaining a flat back throughout the movement
- Pulling into your midriff, not your chest
- Contracting each repetition at the top of the movement

AVOID
- Rounding your back
- Excessively swinging the weight
- Allowing the barbell to drop following the completion of each repetition

BEGINNER MODIFICATION
- Try a lighter resistance.

ADVANCED MODIFICATION
- Try an underhand grip for a fuller range of motion.

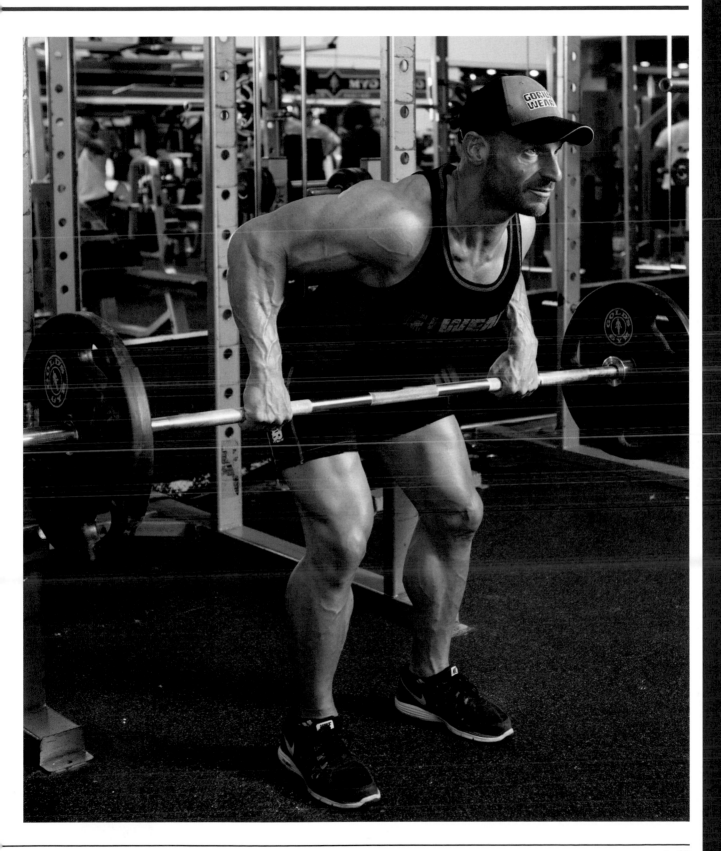

DUMBBELL ROW

PROGRESSION

1 Begin standing above a flat bench with one hand planted and the same-side knee also on the bench.

2 Keep the opposite foot on the ground and a single dumbbell on the same-side hand fully extending downward.

3 While maintaining a flat back, pull the dumbbell up next to your chest, contracting the lat hard.

4 Lower the dumbbell back down to full extension, and then repeat the exercise for 8 to 12 repetitions per side.

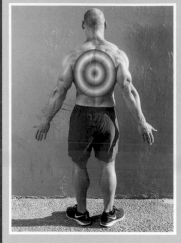

MUSCLE ACTION: PRIMARY ACTIVATION
- upper back
- outer back

ANCILLARY ACTIVATION
- biceps brachii
- rhomboideus
- deltoideus posterior
- forearm extensors
- forearm flexors

PROPER FORM
- Maintaining a flat back throughout the movement
- Pulling next to your chest
- Contracting each repetition at the top of the movement

AVOID
- Rounding your back
- Excessively swinging the weight
- Allowing the dumbbell to drop following the completion of each repetition

BEGINNER MODIFICATION
- Try a lighter resistance.

ADVANCED MODIFICATION
- Try rowing with both arms at the same time without the support from the bench.

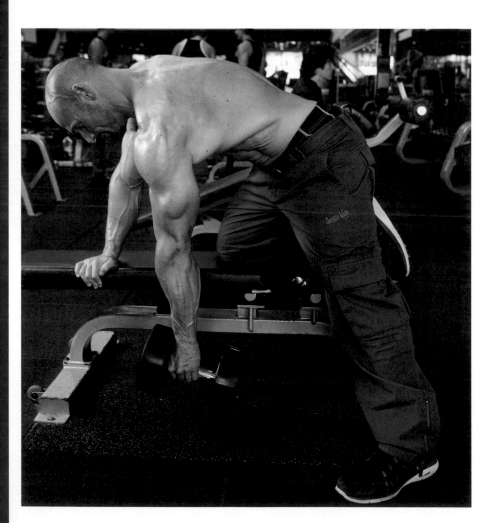

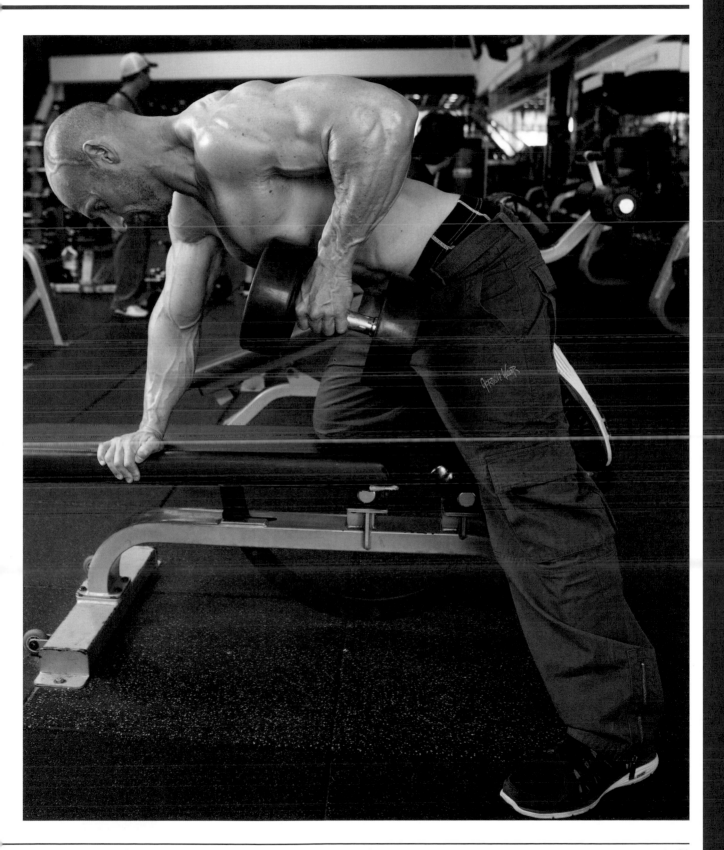

T-BAR ROW

PROGRESSION

1 Begin by standing before a T-Bar Row with your chest against the pad and your feet on the platform.

2 Take a neutral, or palms facing each other, grip, and start by pulling the bar back into your abdomen.

3 Contract the lats at the top of the movement and then return to the starting position for 8 to 12 repetitions.

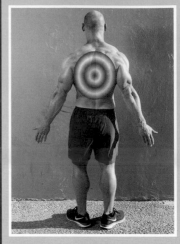

**MUSCLE ACTION:
PRIMARY ACTIVATION**
- upper back
- middle back

ANCILLARY ACTIVATION
- biceps brachii
- rhomboideus
- deltoideus posterior
- forearm extensors
- forearm flexors

PROPER FORM
- Maintaining a flat back throughout the movement
- Pulling into your abdomen, not your chest
- Contracting each repetition at the top of the movement

AVOID
- Rounding your back
- Excessively swinging the weight
- Allowing the weight to drop following the completion of each repetition

BEGINNER MODIFICATION
- Try a lighter resistance.

ADVANCED MODIFICATION
- Try it with a reverse grip.

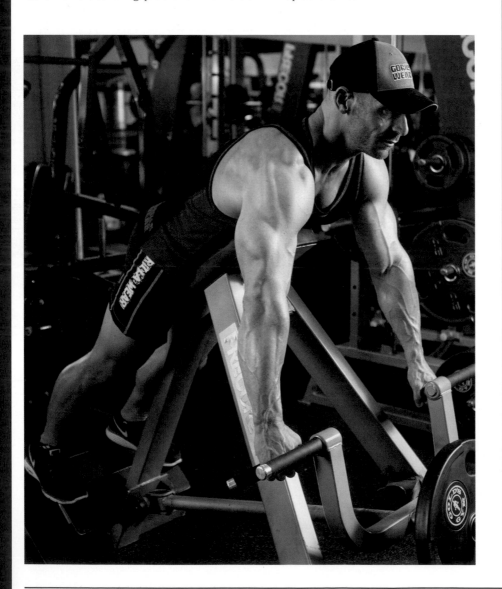

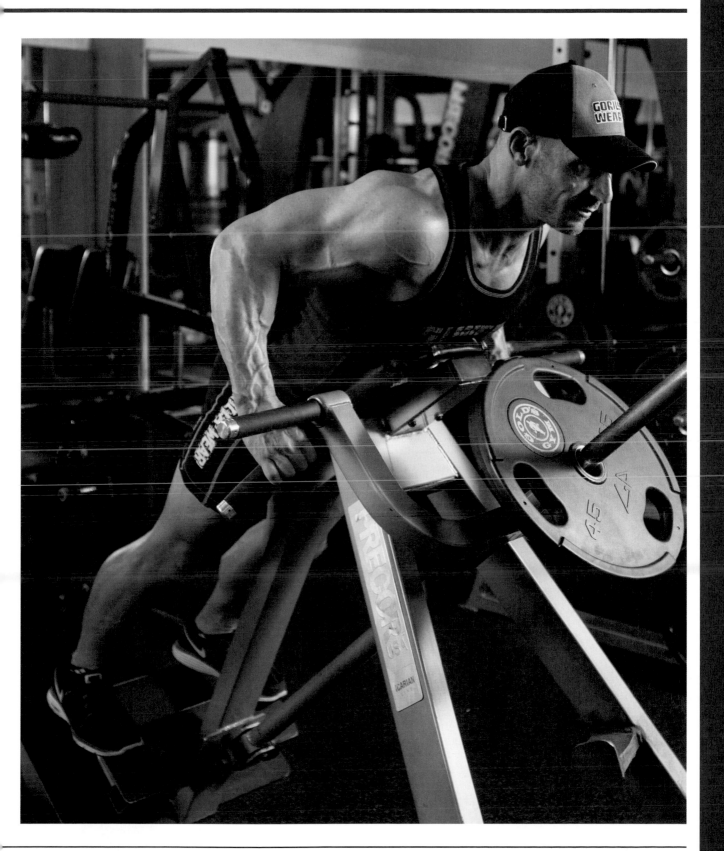

DUMBBELL PULLOVER

PROGRESSION

1 Begin by lying across a flat bench with your shoulders supported and your feet on the floor.

2 Hold a dumbbell above your chest with your hands clasped, your palms upward and your arms fully extended.

3 Start by bending your arms back behind your head, feeling the stretch throughout your upper and outer back.

4 Lengthen your arms as you return the dumbbell to above your chest for 8 to 12 repetitions.

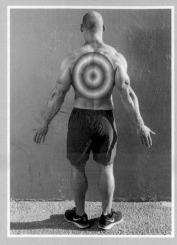

MUSCLE ACTION: PRIMARY ACTIVATION
- latissimus dorsi
- serratus anterior

ANCILLARY ACTIVATION
- triceps brachii
- rectus abdominis

PROPER FORM
- Keeping your pelvis elevated at all times
- Stretching well behind your head
- Bending your arms as you begin the exercise

AVOID
- Dropping your pelvis too low
- Excessively swinging the weight
- Keeping your arms straight as you begin the exercise

BEGINNER MODIFICATION
- Try a lighter resistance.

ADVANCED MODIFICATION
- Try elevating one foot off the ground.

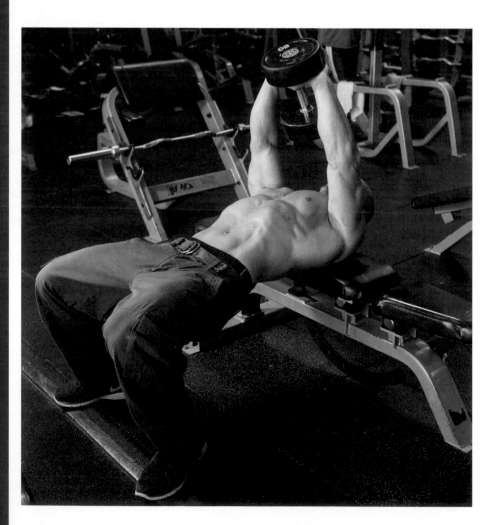

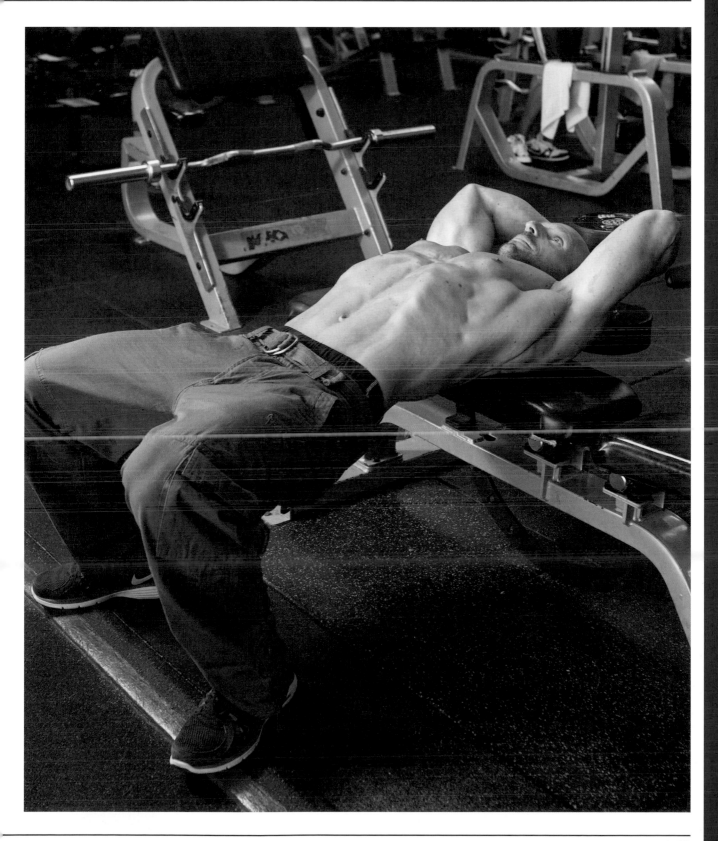

REVERSE HYPEREXTENSION

PROGRESSION

1 Begin standing while facing the side of a stretch table and assume a prone, or facedown, position with your pelvis and legs hanging off the bench.

2 Grip the table with your hands, straighten your legs and keep your feet together.

3 Start by raising your legs, until your body is one straight line and parallel to the ground.

4 Lower and repeat for 12 to 15 repetitions.

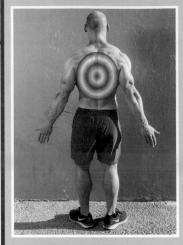

MUSCLE ACTION: PRIMARY ACTIVATION
- erector spinae

ANCILLARY ACTIVATION
- gluteus maximus
- hamstrings

PROPER FORM
- A controlled raising
- Your body situated in a straight line
- Contracting each repetition at the top of the movement

AVOID
- Raising your legs too high
- Excessive swinging movement
- Keeping your pelvis compressed against the table

BEGINNER MODIFICATION
- Try fewer repetitions.

ADVANCED MODIFICATION
- Try it with ankle weights for added resistance.

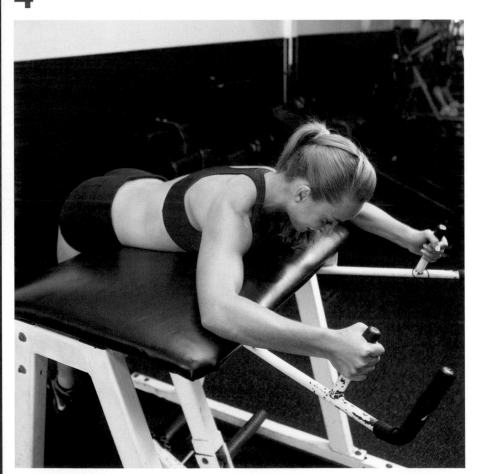

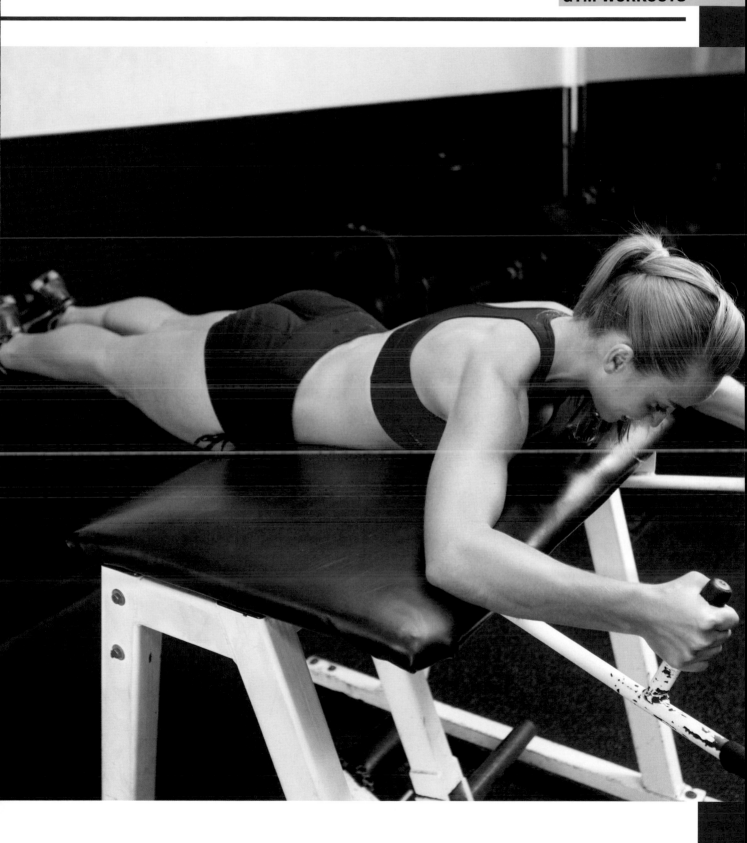

DEADLIFT

PROGRESSION

1 Begin standing in front of a weighted barbell with your feet shoulder-width apart and toes facing forward.

2 Squat down and grab the barbell with a wide overhand grip, positioning your knees close to the bar and keeping your spine straight and your head up.

3 Push through your heels as you stand erect with the barbell held below you at arms' length, and then lower carefully to the ground for 8 to 10 repetitions.

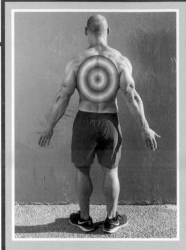

MUSCLE ACTION: PRIMARY ACTIVATION
- erector spinae
- rectus abdominis
- gluteus maximus
- quadriceps
- hamstrings

ANCILLARY ACTIVATION
- trapezius
- biceps brachii
- forearm extensors
- forearm flexors

PROPER FORM
- Maintaining a flat back
- Keeping the bar close to your shins
- Standing completely upright at the top of the movement

AVOID
- Rounding your back
- Excessively slamming the weight down
- Pushing through the toes

BEGINNER MODIFICATION
- Try it with your legs wider and your hands closer.

ADVANCED MODIFICATION
- Vary your foot stance: keeping your feet close together tends to increase the range of motion, making it more difficult.

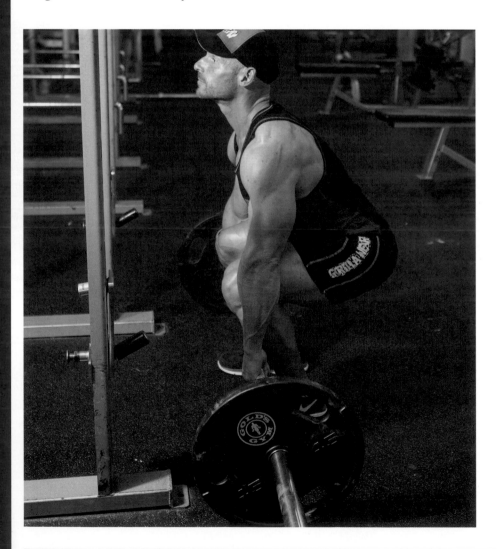

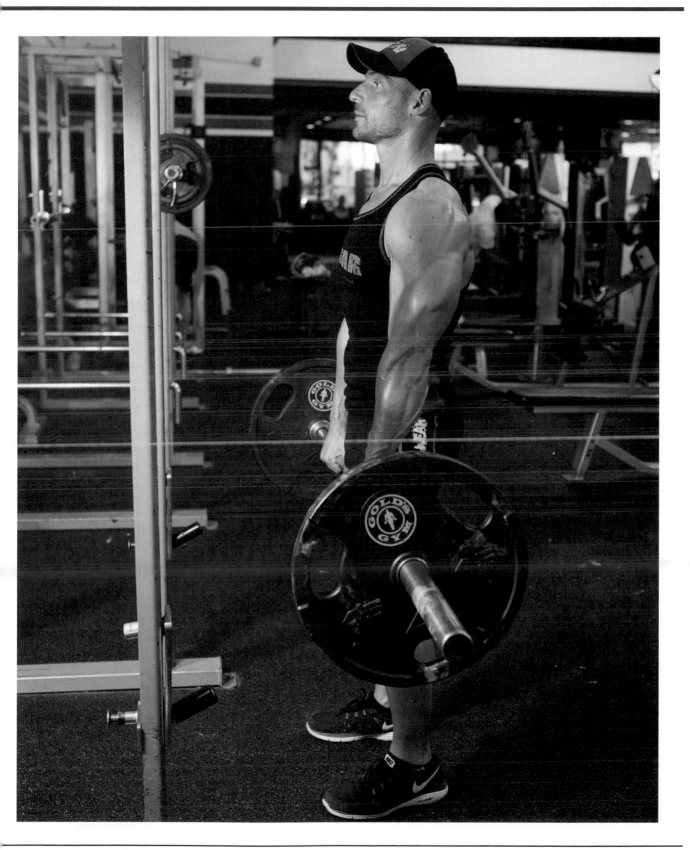

SMITH MACHINE SQUAT

PROGRESSION

1 Begin standing in front of a Smith Machine and duck under the bar, unracking and resting it on the rear of your shoulders.

2 Take a slight step ahead with your feet shoulder-width apart and firmly grip the bar to prevent it from rotating.

3 Bend your knees slightly, sticking your rear out as you bend at the knees, while keeping your back flat and lowering yourself toward the ground until your thighs are parallel to it.

4 Push through your heels to again stand tall, and repeat for 12 to 15 repetitions.

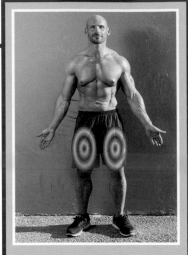

MUSCLE ACTION: PRIMARY ACTIVATION
- quadriceps femoris
- gluteus maximus
- hamstrings

ANCILLARY ACTIVATION
- erector spinae
- transversus abdominis
- hip abductors
- hip adductors
- soleus
- gastrocnemius

PROPER FORM
- Squatting until your thighs are parallel to the ground
- A slow and controlled lowering of the weight
- Pushing through your heels to drive the movement

AVOID
- Hyperextending your knees past your feet
- A rounded back
- A shortened range of motion

BEGINNER MODIFICATION
- Try it with just your body weight.

ADVANCED MODIFICATION
- A closer stance will increase the range of motion.

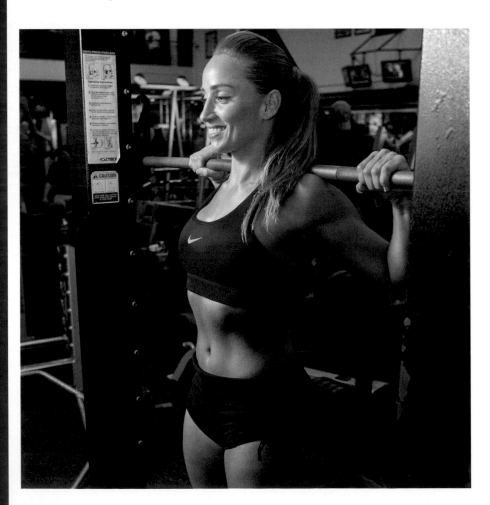

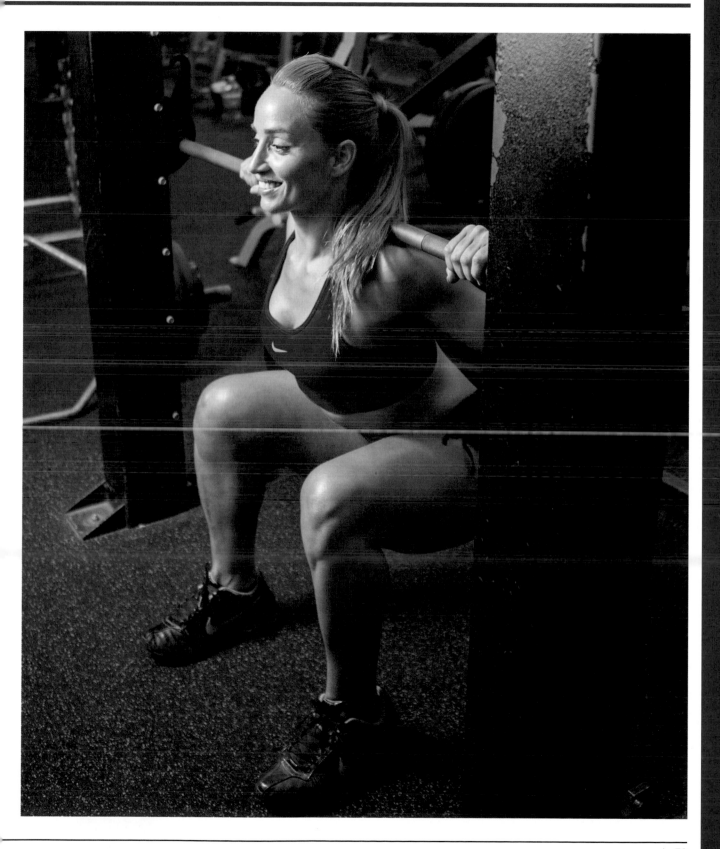

HACK SQUAT

PROGRESSION

1 Begin standing on a Hack Squat platform, with your back against the pad and your feet shoulder-width apart.

2 Release the levers at your sides and start by bending your knees as you lower yourself toward the ground until your thighs are parallel to the platform.

3 Push through your heels to stand tall and repeat for 12 to 15 repetitions.

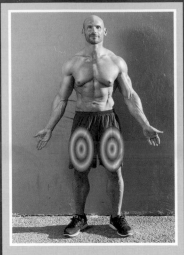

**MUSCLE ACTION:
PRIMARY ACTIVATION**
- quadriceps femoris
- gluteus maximus
- hamstrings

ANCILLARY ACTIVATION
- erector spinae
- transversus abdominis
- hip abductors
- hip adductors
- soleus
- gastrocnemius

PROPER FORM
- Squatting until your thighs are parallel to the ground
- A slow and controlled lowering of the weight
- Pushing through your heels to drive the movement

AVOID
- Hyperextending your knees past your feet
- A crooked descent
- A shortened range of motion

BEGINNER MODIFICATION
- Try it with a wider stance.

ADVANCED MODIFICATION
- Try it with a closer stance.

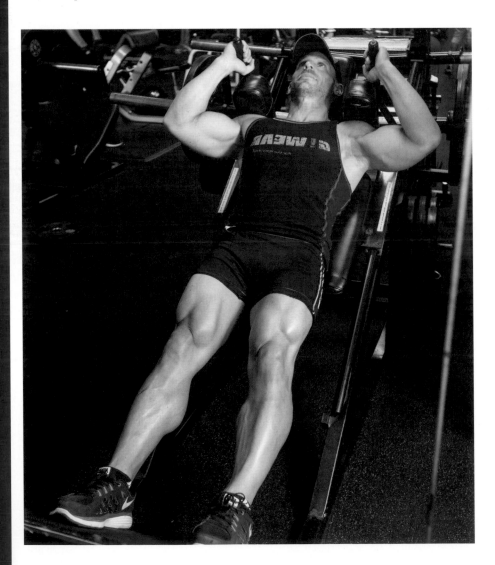

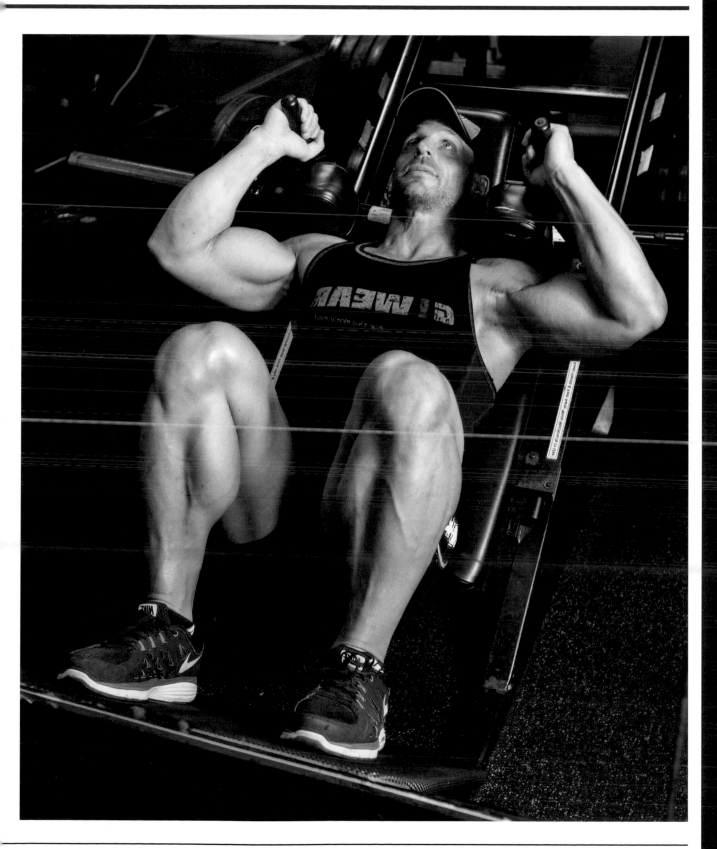

LEG PRESS

PROGRESSION

1 Begin seated with your back against the pad of a Leg Press Machine and your feet placed less than shoulder-width apart on the foot placement board.

2 Unrack the weight as you lower the sled toward your chest to a 90-degree angle, then drive the weight up to full extension by pushing through your heels for 12 to 15 repetitions.

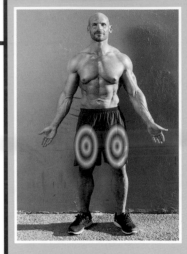

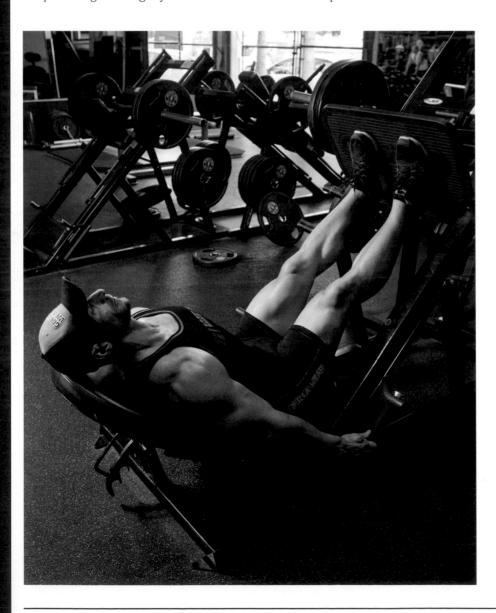

MUSCLE ACTION:
PRIMARY ACTIVATION
- quadriceps femoris
- gluteus maximus
- hamstrings

ANCILLARY ACTIVATION
- rectus abdominis
- soleus
- gastrocnemius

PROPER FORM
- Pushing through the heels to drive the exercise
- Keeping your feet in line with your knees
- Performing a full range of motion

AVOID
- Pushing through your toes
- Wearing a weight belt
- Allowing your lower back and butt to come up

BEGINNER MODIFICATION
- A wider foot placement will decrease your range of motion.

ADVANCED MODIFICATION
- Try it with one leg for a greater challenge.

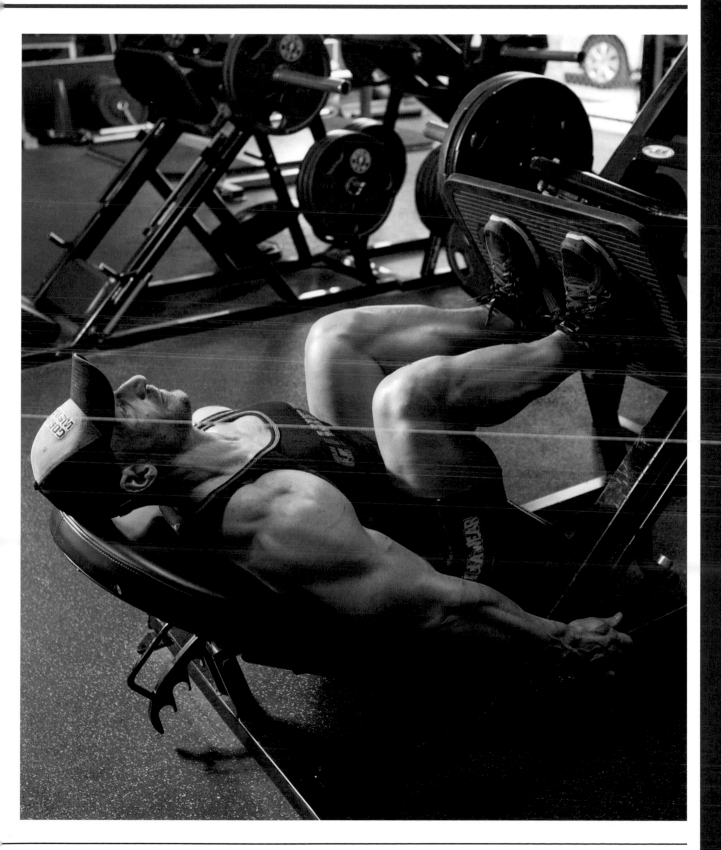

ALTERNATE REVERSE LUNGE

PROGRESSION

1 Begin in a standing position while holding a pair of dumbbells at your sides and start by taking one giant step back with one leg, bending both legs until the front thigh is parallel to the ground and the back heel is up.

2 Push through your front heel as you return your rear leg to the starting position, standing tall, and then alternating legs for 12 to 15 repetitions per leg.

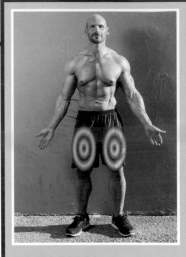

**MUSCLE ACTION:
PRIMARY ACTIVATION**
- quadriceps femoris
- gluteus maximus
- hamstrings

ANCILLARY ACTIVATION
- erector spinae
- transversus abdominis
- hip abductors
- hip adductors
- soleus
- gastrocnemius

PROPER FORM
- Pushing through the front heel to drive the movement
- Lunging until your front thigh is parallel to the ground
- Allowing the rear heel to rise

AVOID
- Allowing the knee to hyperextend past the front foot
- Keeping the rear heel flat
- A slouched posture

BEGINNER MODIFICATION
- Try using just your body weight.

ADVANCED MODIFICATION
- Try it with a barbell across your rear shoulders.

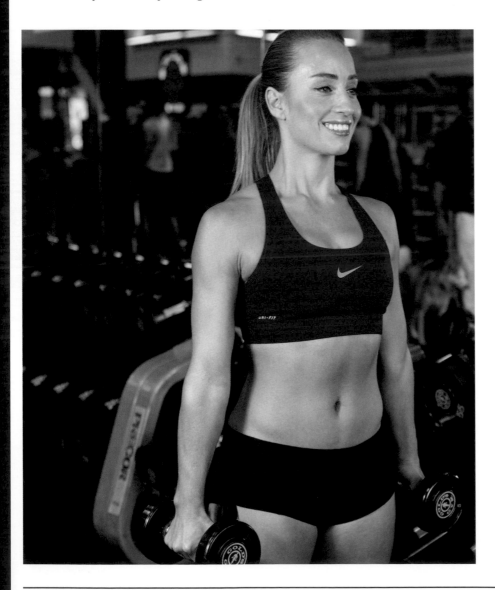

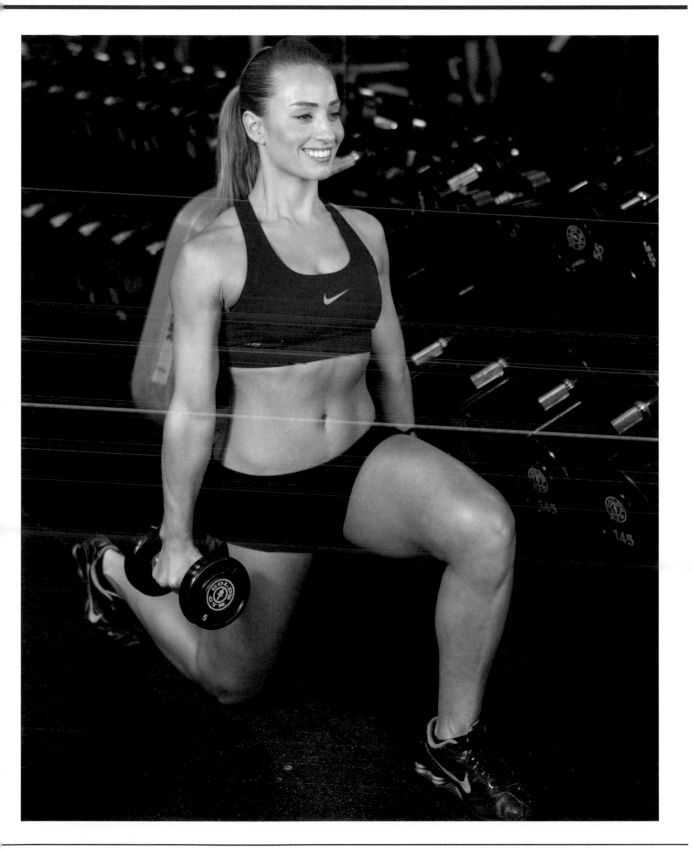

LEG EXTENSION

PROGRESSION

1 Begin in a seated position on a Leg Extension Machine with your back braced against the pad and your lower legs positioned behind the rollers.

2 Keeping your hands on the grips at your sides, extend your lower legs upward, until your legs are in one straight line.

3 Lower back down slowly to the starting position, and then repeat for 12 to 15 controlled repetitions.

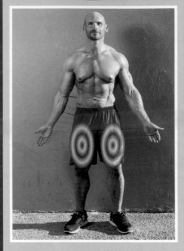

**MUSCLE ACTION:
PRIMARY ACTIVATION**
- quadriceps femoris

ANCILLARY ACTIVATION
- rectus abdominis
- tibialis anterior

PROPER FORM
- A controlled downward range of motion
- Pointing the toes forward during the movement should knee pain persist
- A proper contraction at the top of the movement

AVOID
- Speedy or bouncy repetitions
- Allowing the downward portion of the repetition to crash
- Leaning too far forward to cheat the weight up

BEGINNER MODIFICATION
- Try using a lighter weight.

ADVANCED MODIFICATION
- Try it one leg at a time.

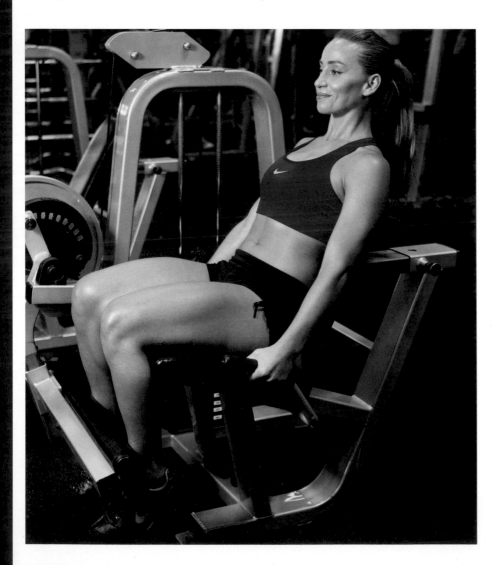

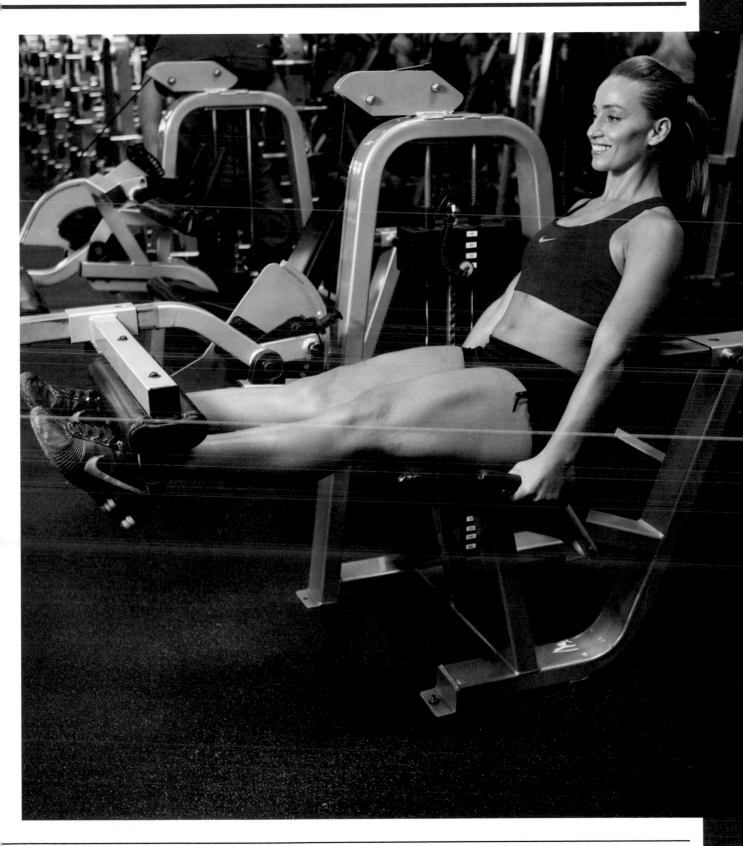

LYING LEG CURL

PROGRESSION

1 Begin by lying face down on a Leg Curl Machine with your lower legs under the rollers, your knees hanging off the bench and your hands on the grips in front of you.

2 Start by bending your legs back at the knees until fully contracted at the top, nearest the gluteal muscles.

3 Lower back down in a controlled manner to lengthen the muscle, and repeat for 10 to 12 repetitions.

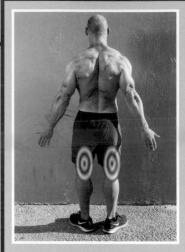

MUSCLE ACTION: PRIMARY ACTIVATION
- hamstrings
- gluteus maximus

ANCILLARY ACTIVATION
- erector spinae
- gastrocnemius

PROPER FORM
- A controlled downward range of motion
- Pointing the toes forward during the movement should knee pain persist
- A proper contraction at the top of the movement

AVOID
- Speedy repetitions
- A short range of motion
- Leaning your upper body backward to cheat the weight up

BEGINNER MODIFICATION
- Try using a lighter weight.

ADVANCED MODIFICATION
- Try it one leg at a time.

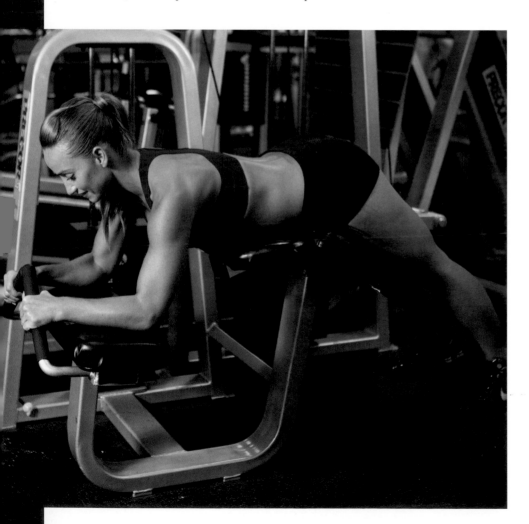

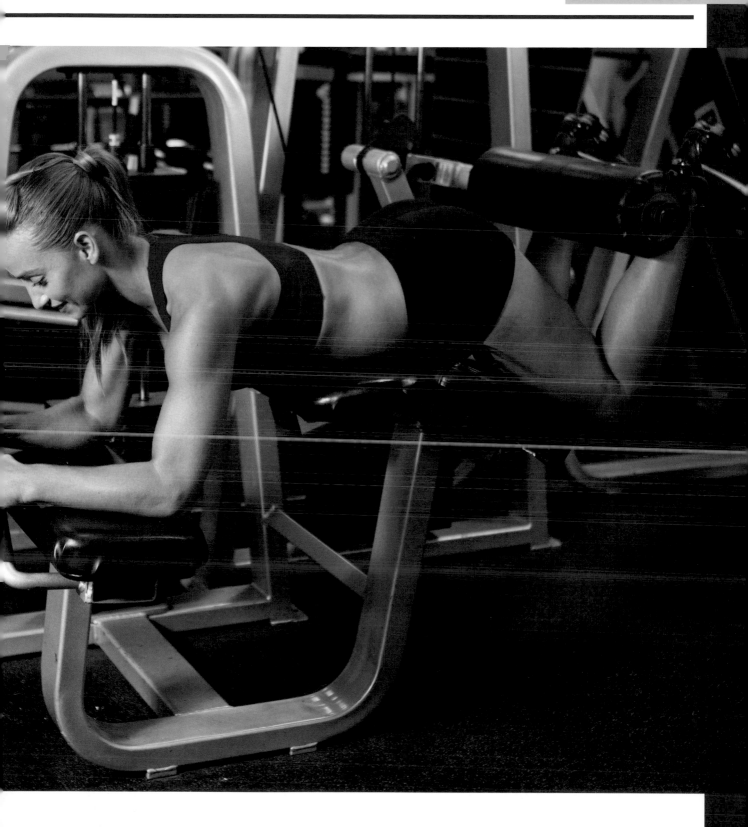

SEATED LEG CURL

PROGRESSION

1 Begin seated in a Leg Curl Machine with your legs fully extended in front of you, your calves resting on the pads and your body firmly locked in place.

2 Bend your legs down and back at the knee, until fully contracted in the flexed position.

3 Slowly extend your legs back up to the starting position to lengthen the muscle, and repeat for 12 to 15 repetitions.

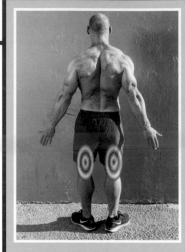

MUSCLE ACTION: PRIMARY ACTIVATION
- hamstrings
- gluteus maximus

ANCILLARY ACTIVATION
- rectus abdominis
- gastrocnemius

PROPER FORM
- A controlled range of motion
- A full contraction in the flexed position
- A full extension at the beginning of the exercise

AVOID
- Speedy repetitions
- A short range of motion
- Leaning your upper body forward to cheat the weight up

BEGINNER MODIFICATION
- Try using a lighter weight.

ADVANCED MODIFICATION
- Try holding the contracted position longer.

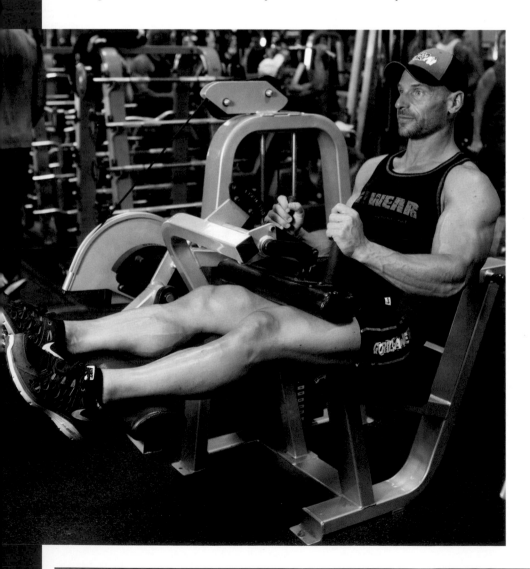

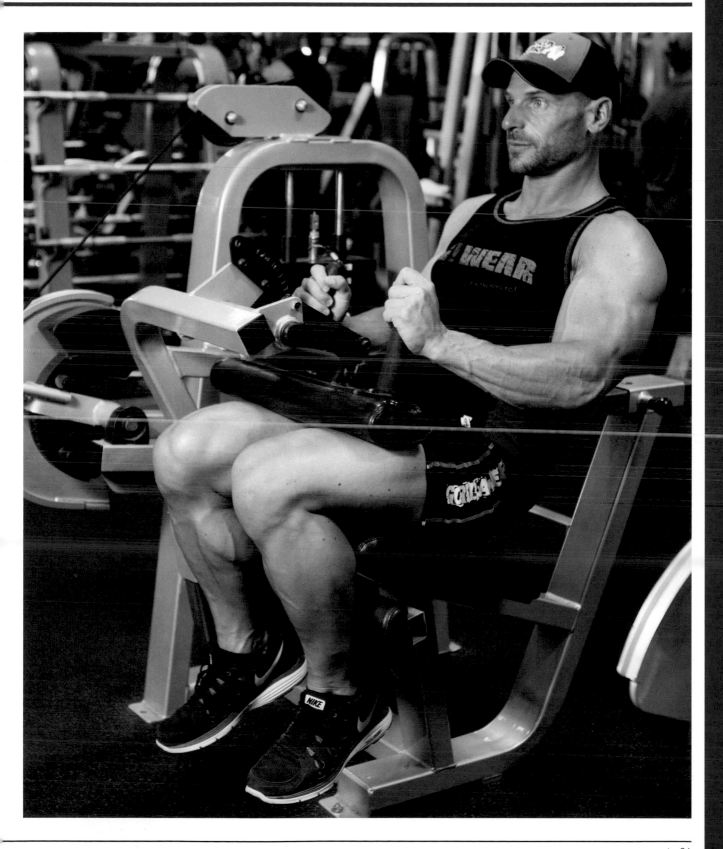

ONE-LEGGED CURL

PROGRESSION

1 Begin by standing in front of a Leg Curl Machine with one leg placed in front of the roller and the other off to the side, with both hands on the grips in front of you.

2 Bend the working leg back and upward in a curling motion until fully contracted at the top nearest the gluteal muscles.

3 Slowly lower back down in a controlled manner to lengthen the muscle, and repeat for 12 to 15 repetitions per leg.

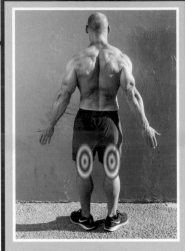

**MUSCLE ACTION:
PRIMARY ACTIVATION**
- hamstrings
- gluteus maximus

ANCILLARY ACTIVATION
- gastrocnemius
- erector spinae

PROPER FORM
- A controlled range of motion
- A full contraction in the flexed position
- A full extension at the beginning of the exercise

AVOID
- Speedy repetitions
- A short range of motion
- Leaning your upper body forward to cheat the weight up

BEGINNER MODIFICATION
- Try using a lighter weight.

ADVANCED MODIFICATION
- Try holding the contracted position longer.

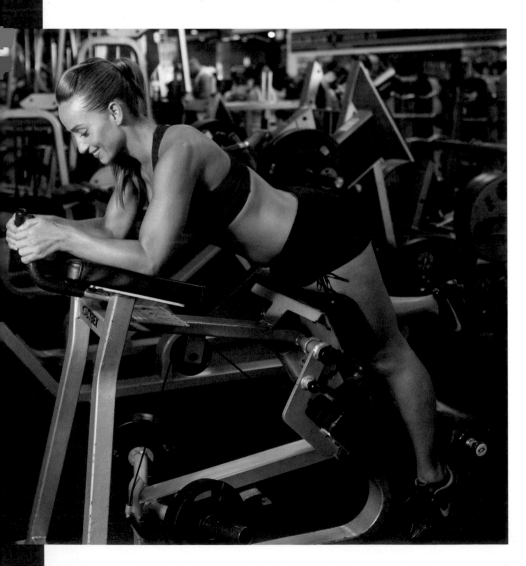

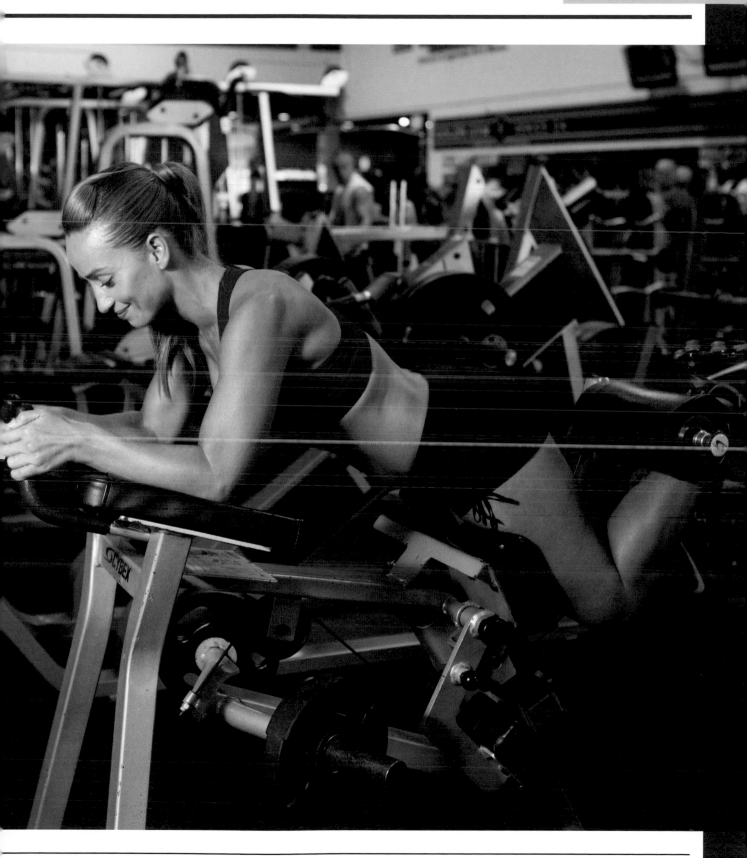

STANDING CALF RAISES

PROGRESSION

1 Begin by ducking under the shoulder pads of a Standing Calf Raise Machine with your body in a straight line, your knees soft and your toes placed on the edge of the foot platform.

2 Rise up on your toes, contracting your calf muscles at the top, and then lower back down past the platform for a full stretch for 12 to 15 repetitions.

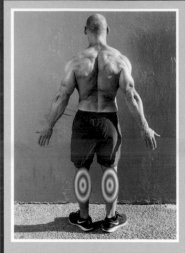

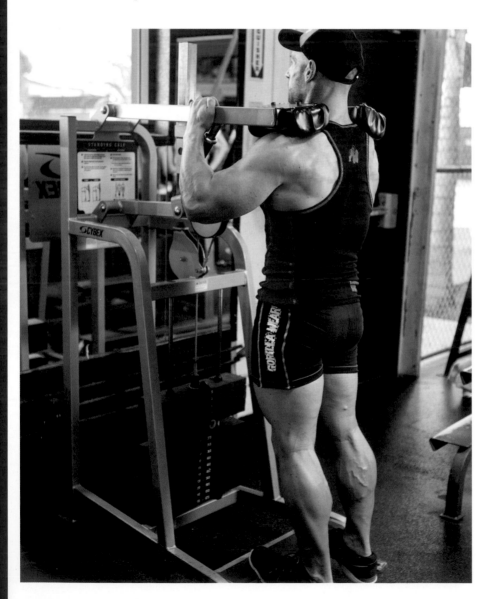

MUSCLE ACTION: PRIMARY ACTIVATION
- gastrocnemius
- soleus

ANCILLARY ACTIVATION
- tibialis anterior

PROPER FORM
- Maintaining a full range of motion
- Contracting your muscles at the top of the movement
- Keeping your toes pointed straight on

AVOID
- Partial repetitions
- Bouncy and speedy repetitions
- Excessively bending your legs

BEGINNER MODIFICATION
- Try using just your body weight.

ADVANCED MODIFICATION
- Try it one calf at a time.

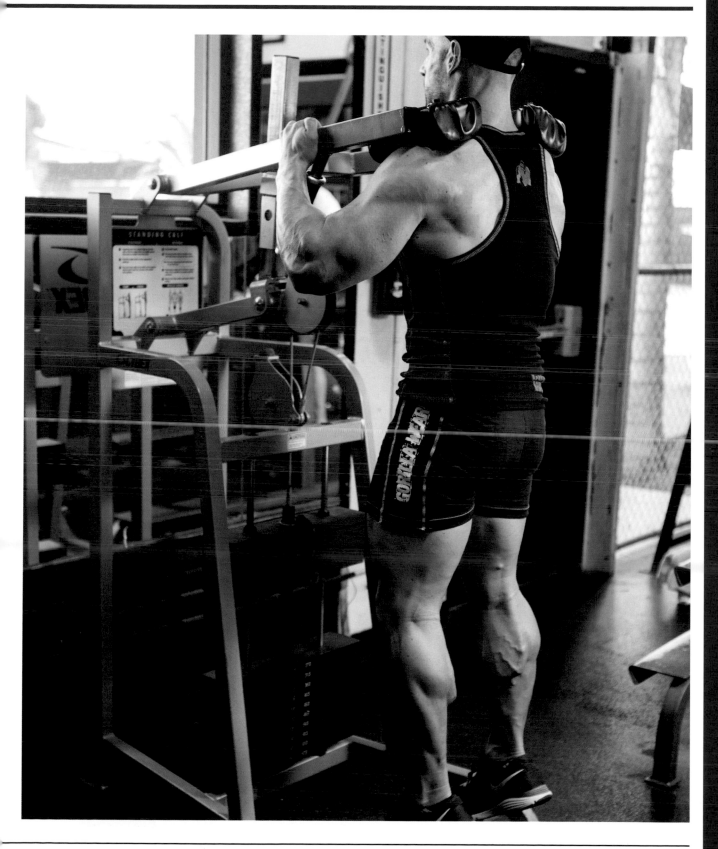

SEATED DUMBBELL PRESS

PROGRESSION

1 Begin in a seated position holding a pair of dumbbells at the level of your outer shoulders with your palms facing forward.

2 Press upward and inward in an arc so that the dumbbells are nearly touching at the top, and then lower them along the same pathway, and repeat for 8 to 12 repetitions.

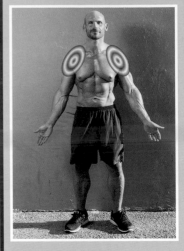

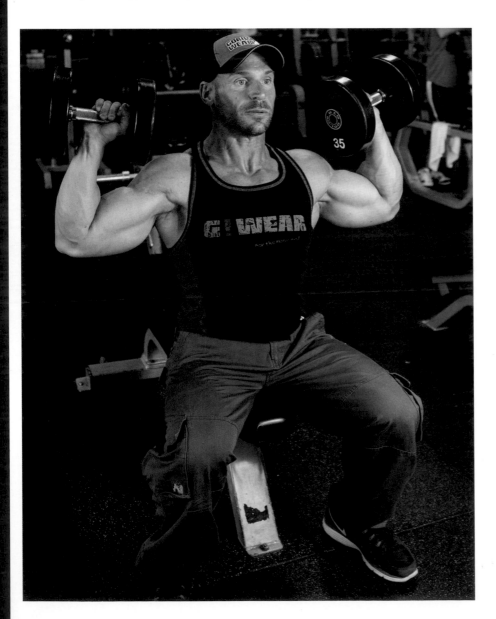

MUSCLE ACTION: PRIMARY ACTIVATION
- deltoideus anterior

ANCILLARY ACTIVATION
- deltoideus medialis
- triceps brachii
- trapezius
- rhomboideus
- rectus abdominis
- erector spinae

PROPER FORM
- Slow and controlled repetitions
- Keeping your torso stabilized and your back pressed against the pad
- Lowering toward your outer shoulders

AVOID
- Keeping your back away from the pad
- Lowering too far inside the shoulders
- Lacking a full range of motion

BEGINNER MODIFICATION
- Try it with a barbell.

ADVANCED MODIFICATION
- Try alternating arms.

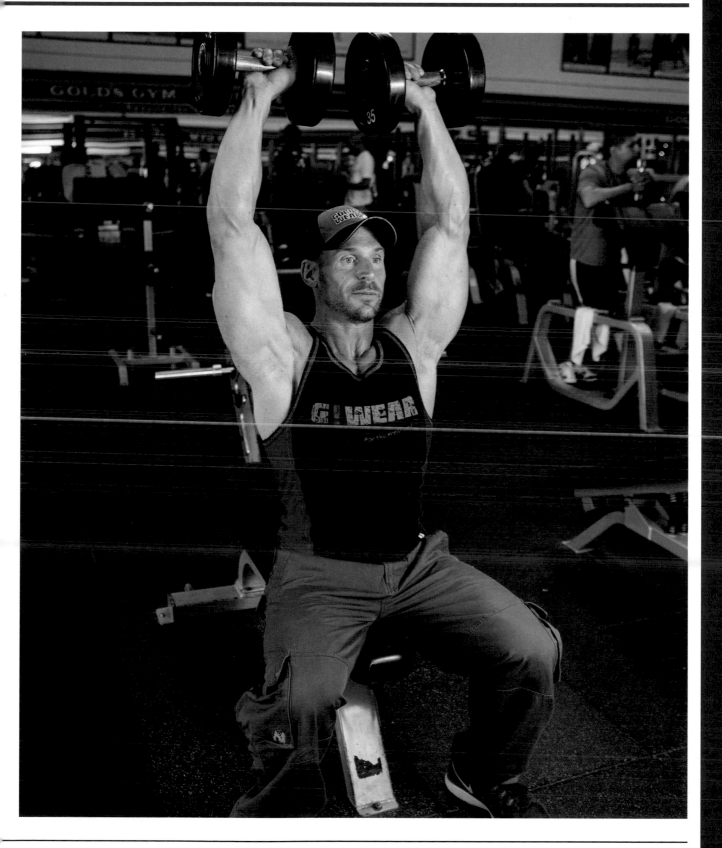

FRONT BARBELL RAISE

PROGRESSION

1 Begin in a standing position while holding a barbell directly below you at arms' length with an overhand grip and your hands shoulder-width apart.

2 While keeping your arms slightly bent, start by raising the barbell upward and away from you until your arms are parallel to the ground.

3 Lower and repeat for 10 to 12 repetitions.

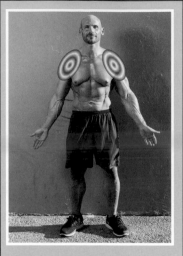

**MUSCLE ACTION:
PRIMARY ACTIVATION**
- deltoideus anterior

ANCILLARY ACTIVATION
- deltoideus medialis
- triceps brachii
- trapezius
- rhomboideus
- rectus abdominis
- erector spinae

PROPER FORM
- Maintaining posture throughout the exercise
- Keeping your arms slightly bent throughout the movement
- A controlled lowering of the weight

AVOID
- Excessive speed or momentum
- Leaning backward
- Keeping your arms straight

BEGINNER MODIFICATION
- Try it with a lighter weight.

ADVANCED MODIFICATION
- Try it alternating your arms with dumbbells.

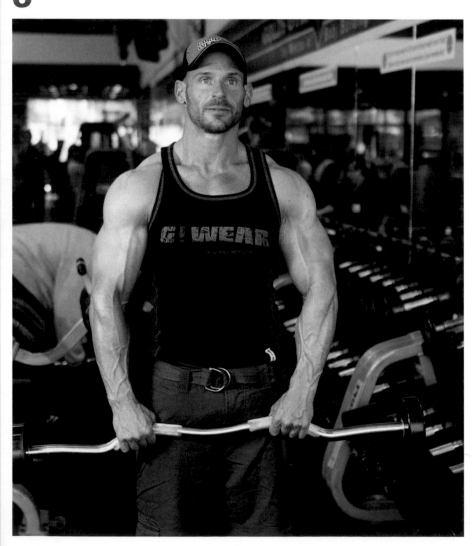

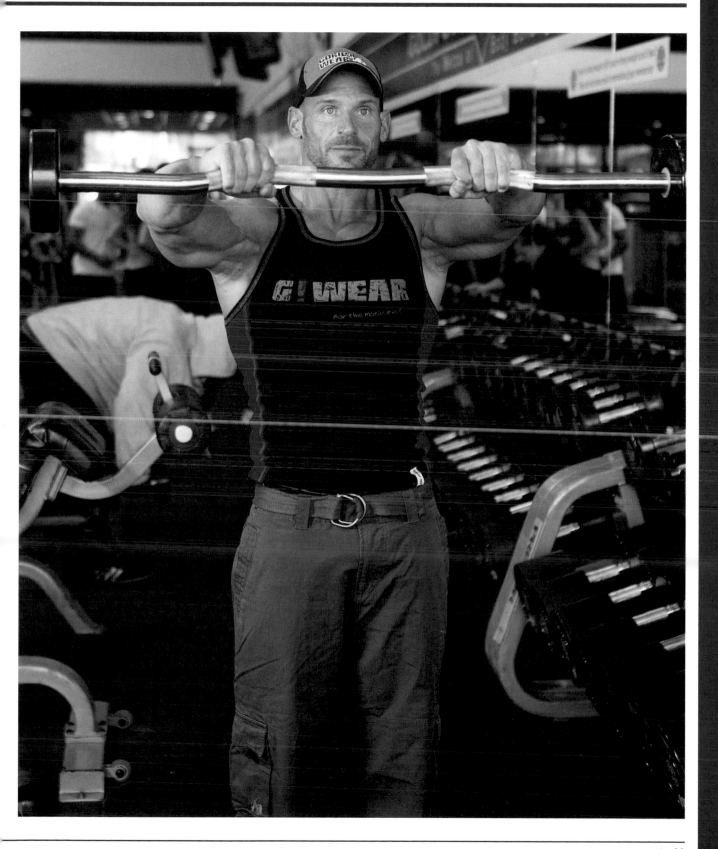

STANDING LATERAL RAISE

PROGRESSION

1 Begin in a standing position holding a pair of dumbbells with your palms facing inward.

2 Start by raising your arms directly out to the sides, with slightly bent arms, turning your thumbs slightly downward as you raise your arms parallel to the ground.

3 Lower and repeat for 10 to 12 repetitions.

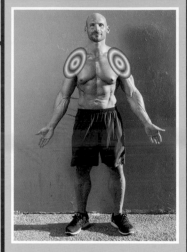

**MUSCLE ACTION:
PRIMARY ACTIVATION**
- deltoideus medialis

ANCILLARY ACTIVATION
- trapezius
- rhomboideus
- forearm flexors
- forearm extensors

PROPER FORM
- Maintaining proper posture throughout the exercise
- Keeping your arms slightly bent throughout the movement
- Your thumbs pointed slightly downward as you raise your arms

AVOID
- Raising your arms above parallel to the ground
- Excessive speed or momentum
- Allowing the anterior deltoids to take over the movement

BEGINNER MODIFICATION
- Try it with a lighter weight.

ADVANCED MODIFICATION
- Try alternating arms.

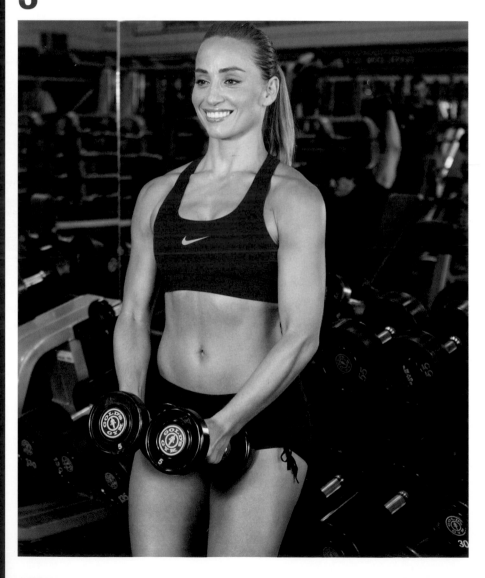

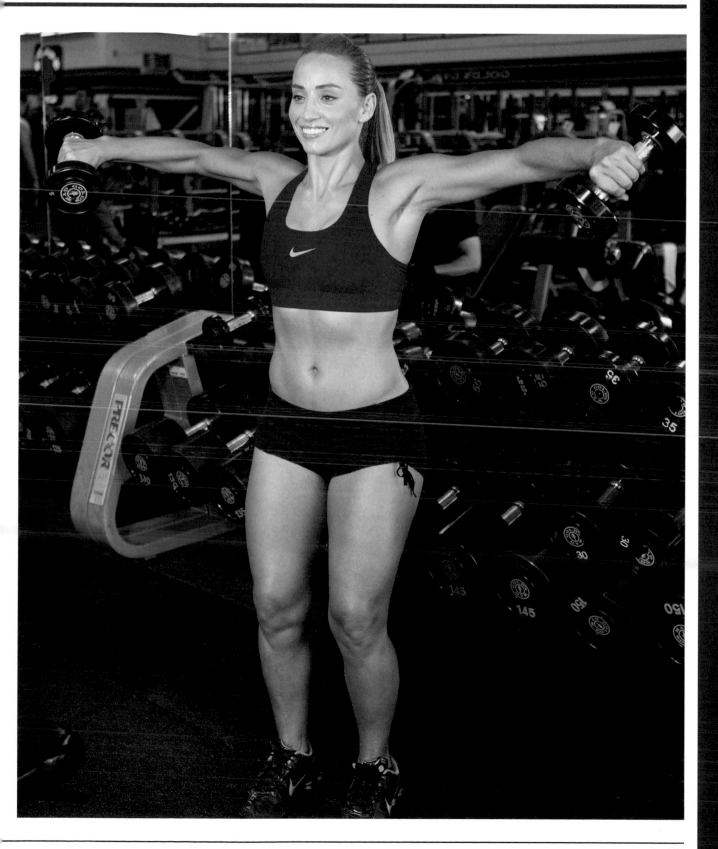

REVERSE FLYE

PROGRESSION

1 Begin seated in a Rear Deltoid Machine facing the pad, or inward, with your hands gripping the handles in front of you.

2 Start by bending your arms directly out to the sides, with slightly bent arms, in a reverse hugging motion.

3 Return and repeat for 10 to 12 repetitions.

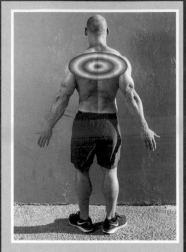

MUSCLE ACTION: PRIMARY ACTIVATION
- deltoideus posterior

ANCILLARY ACTIVATION
- trapezius
- rhomboideus
- forearm flexors
- forearm extensors

PROPER FORM
- Keeping your chest braced against the pad throughout the movement
- Keeping your arms slightly bent throughout the movement
- A reverse hugging motion

AVOID
- Excessive speed or momentum
- Leaning excessively backward
- Keeping your arms straight

BEGINNER MODIFICATION
- Try it with a lighter weight.

ADVANCED MODIFICATION
- Try alternating arms.

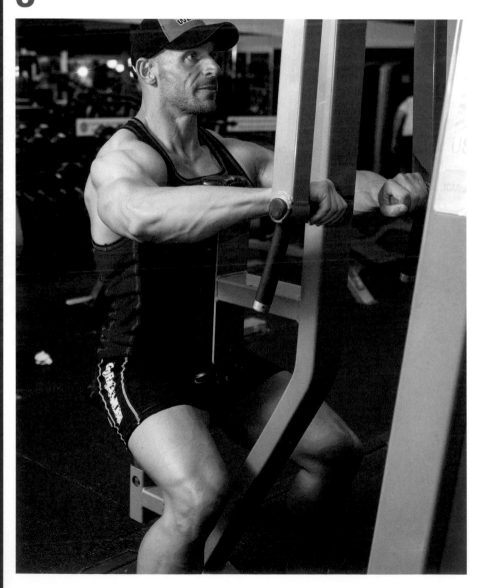

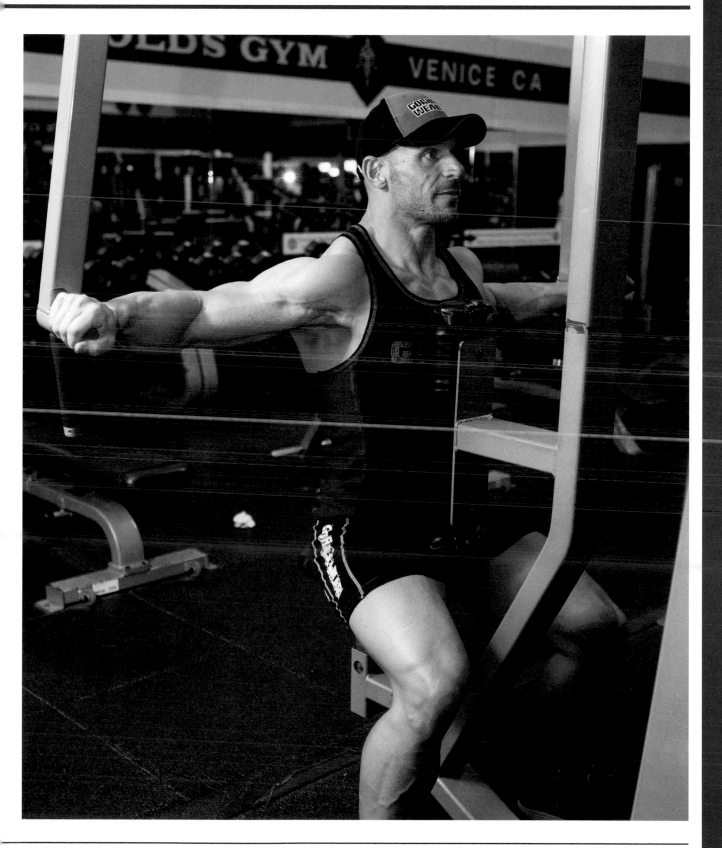

UPRIGHT ROW

PROGRESSION

1 Begin in a standing position holding a barbell below you at arms' length with an overhand grip spaced a few inches apart.

2 Pull the barbell straight up to chin level while leading with your elbows. Lower and repeat for 10 to 12 repetitions.

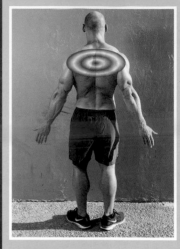

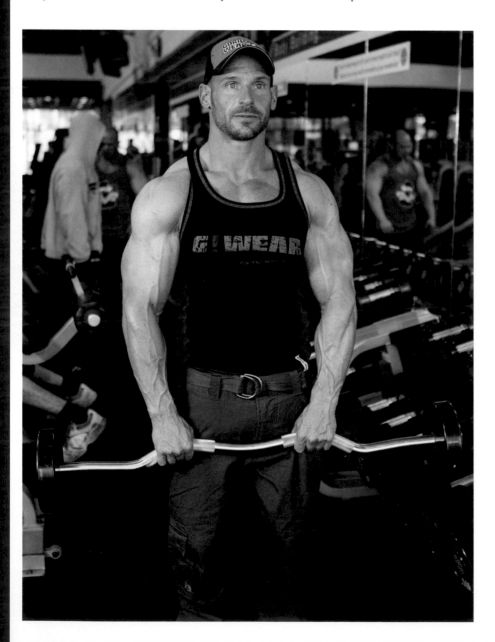

MUSCLE ACTION: PRIMARY ACTIVATION
- deltoideus medialis
- trapezius

ANCILLARY ACTIVATION
- rhomboideus
- biceps brachii
- forearm flexors
- forearm extensors

PROPER FORM
- Keeping the barbell close to your body
- Leading with the elbows
- Raising no higher than chin level

AVOID
- Excessive speed or momentum
- Allowing your elbows to drop
- Pulling the barbell away from the body

BEGINNER MODIFICATION
- Try using a closer grip.

ADVANCED MODIFICATION
- Try it with dumbbells.

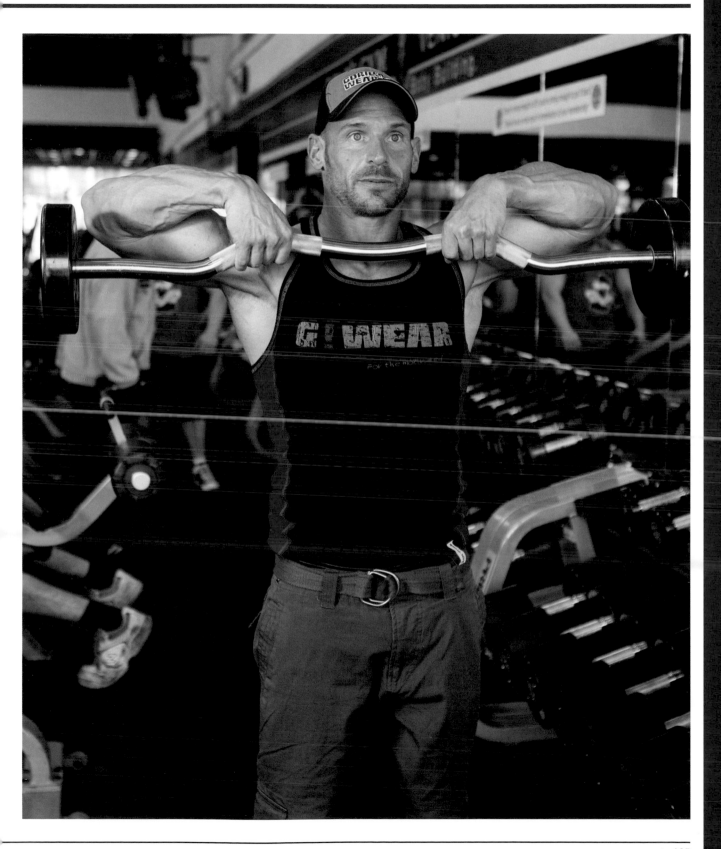

STANDING ALTERNATE DUMBBELL CURL

PROGRESSION

1 Begin by standing with a pair of dumbbells at arms' length at your sides with your palms facing each other.

2 Start the movement by bending one arm at a time at the elbow, while simultaneously supinating, or turning your palm upward, until your hand is nearly touching your shoulder.

3 Pronate, or turn the palm outward, as you return to the starting position while bringing the other arm up for 10 to 12 repetitions per arm.

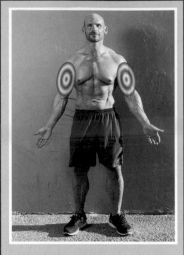

MUSCLE ACTION: PRIMARY ACTIVATION
- biceps brachii

ANCILLARY ACTIVATION
- rectus abdominis
- erector spinae
- forearm flexors
- forearm extensors

PROPER FORM
- A full and complete range of motion
- Elbows close to your body throughout the movement
- A controlled lowering of the weight

AVOID
- Swinging the weight up
- Excessive speed or momentum
- Using your lower back excessively

BEGINNER MODIFICATION
- Try using a lighter weight.

ADVANCED MODIFICATION
- Try it with both arms at the same time.

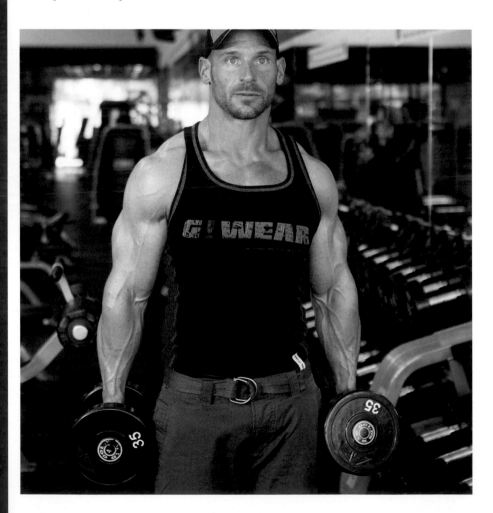

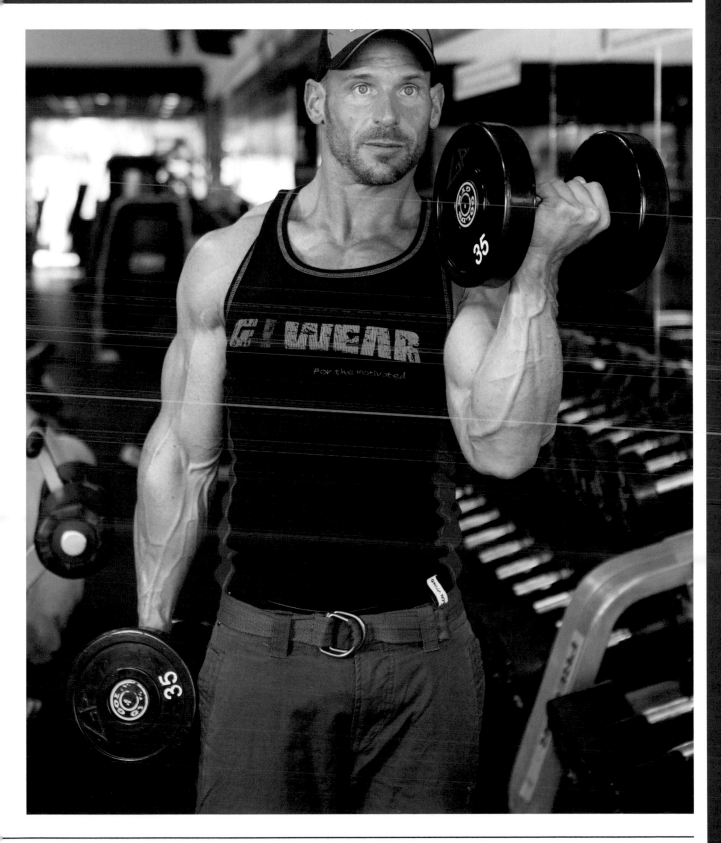

ROPE HAMMER CURL

PROGRESSION

1 Begin by standing in front of a cable stack holding a rope attachment with a thumbs-up grip at arm's length with your palms facing each other.

2 While keeping the rope split apart, bend at the elbows until your hands are nearly touching your shoulders.

3 Lower the rope, and return to the starting position for 10 to 12 repetitions.

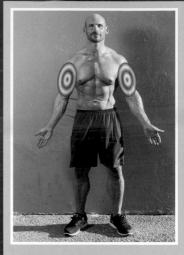

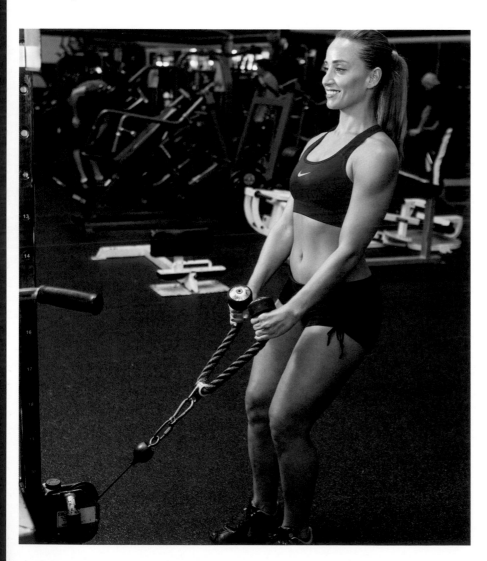

MUSCLE ACTION: PRIMARY ACTIVATION
- biceps brachii
- brachialis

ANCILLARY ACTIVATION
- rectus abdominis
- erector spinae
- forearm flexors
- forearm extensors

PROPER FORM
- Thumbs up throughout the movement
- Your elbows close to your body
- A controlled lowering of the weight

AVOID
- Swinging the weight up
- Excessive speed or momentum
- Using your lower back excessively

BEGINNER MODIFICATION
- Try using a lighter weight.

ADVANCED MODIFICATION
- Try it with dumbbells.

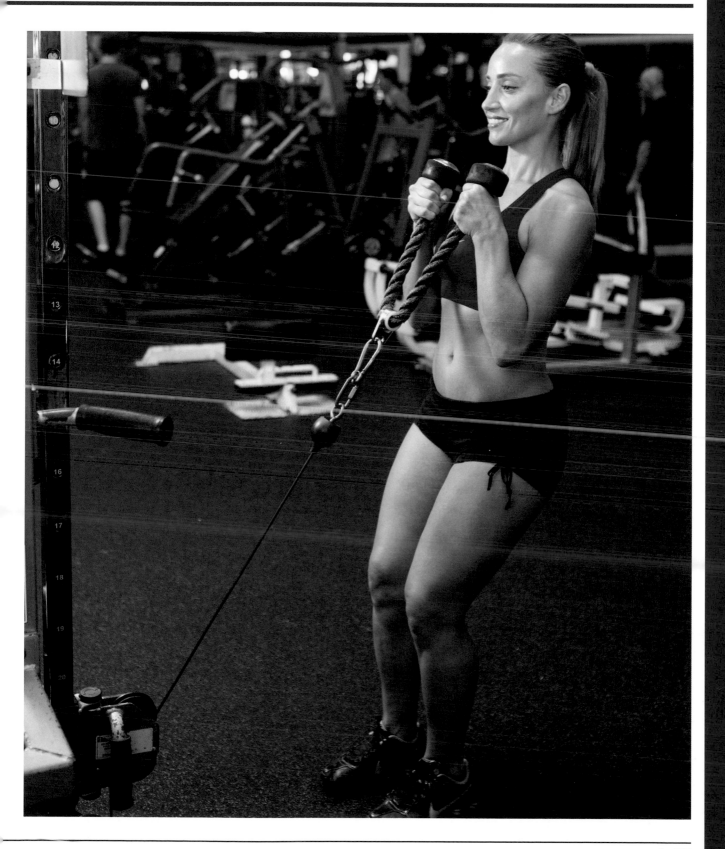

PREACHER CURL

PROGRESSION

1 Begin sitting at a Preacher Curl Machine with an underhand, shoulder-width grip on the handles held at arms' length in front of you.

2 Start the movement by bending at the elbows, until your palms are nearly touching your shoulders.

3 Lower your arms, and return to the starting position for 10 to 12 repetitions.

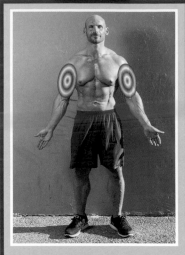

**MUSCLE ACTION:
PRIMARY ACTIVATION**
- biceps brachii

ANCILLARY ACTIVATION
- rectus abdominis
- erector spinae
- forearm flexors
- forearm extensors

PROPER FORM
- A full and complete range of motion
- Keeping your elbows in
- A controlled lowering of the weight

AVOID
- Allowing your upper arms to lift off the bench
- Excessive speed or momentum
- Using your shoulders excessively

BEGINNER MODIFICATION
- Try a lighter weight.

ADVANCED MODIFICATION
- Try it with a dumbbell.

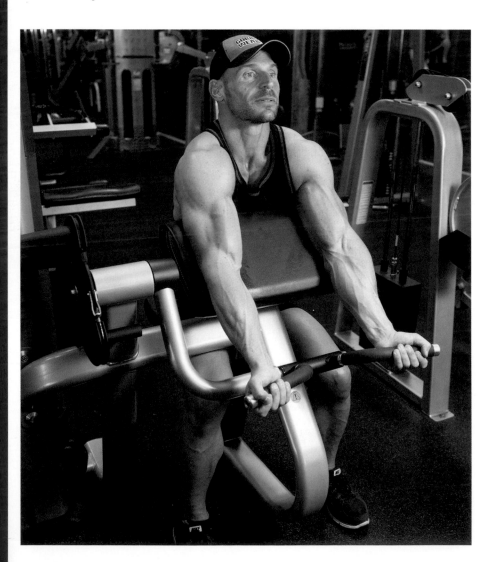

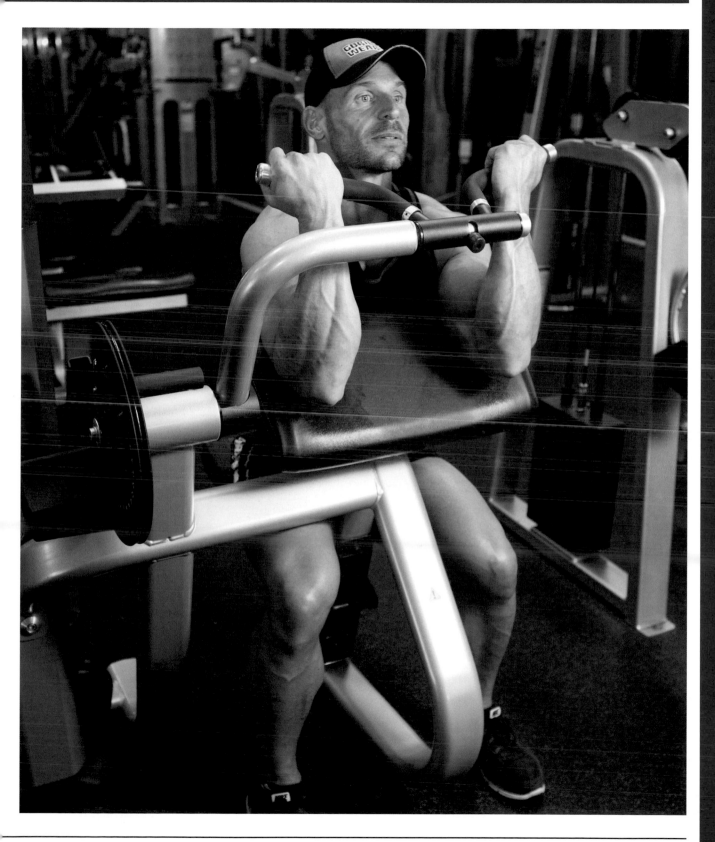

ONE-ARM CABLE CURL

PROGRESSION

1 Begin by standing in front of a pulley stack with the cable set at the low position and holding one handle with an underhand grip positioned at arm's length in front of you and your palm facing your thigh.

2 Start the movement by simultaneously bending your arm at the elbow and turning your wrist upward until your palm is facing upward and nearly touching your shoulder.

3 Return to the starting position by both lengthening your arm and turning your wrist outward for 12 to 15 repetitions on each arm.

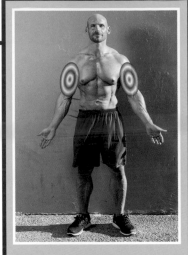

**MUSCLE ACTION:
PRIMARY ACTIVATION**
• biceps brachii

ANCILLARY ACTIVATION
• forearm flexors
• forearm extensors

PROPER FORM
• A full and complete range of motion
• Proper body posture and alignment
• A controlled lowering of the weight

AVOID
• Swinging the weight up
• Excessive speed or momentum
• Using your lower back excessively

BEGINNER MODIFICATION
• Try using a lighter weight.

ADVANCED MODIFICATION
• Try it with dumbbells.

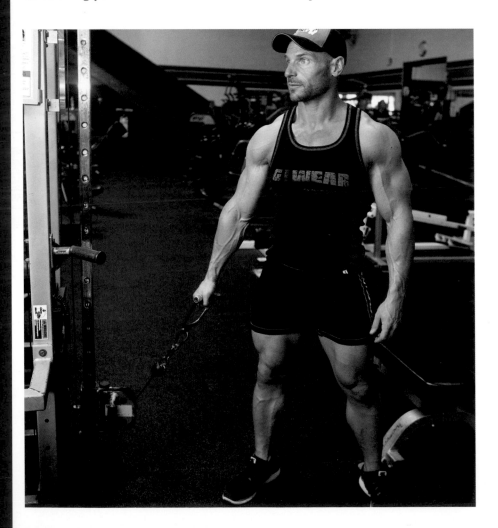

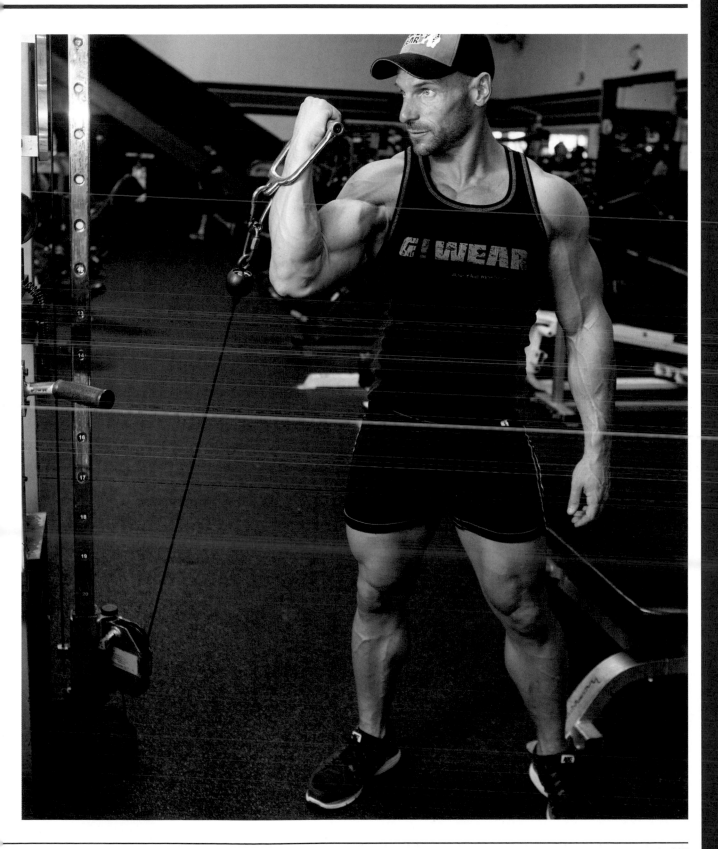

LYING TRICEPS EXTENSION

PROGRESSION

1 Begin by lying on your back on a flat bench with an inside, overhand grip on a cambered bar and your feet on the ground.

2 Start with the bar above your chest with your arms extended to full lockout, and then bend your arms backward at the elbow, past your head.

3 Keeping your elbows in and locked in place, extend the bar back up to full lockout over your chest and repeat for 10 to 12 repetitions.

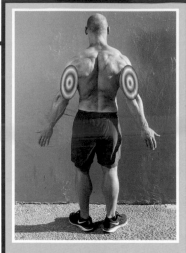

MUSCLE ACTION: PRIMARY ACTIVATION
• triceps brachii

ANCILLARY ACTIVATION
• deltoideus anterior
• rectus abdominis

PROPER FORM
• A full stretch behind your head
• Keeping your torso stabilized and your upper body straight
• Keeping your elbows in

AVOID
• Excessive speed
• Knocking yourself in the head
• Flared elbows

BEGINNER MODIFICATION
• Try it with a lighter weight.

ADVANCED MODIFICATION
• Try it with dumbbells.

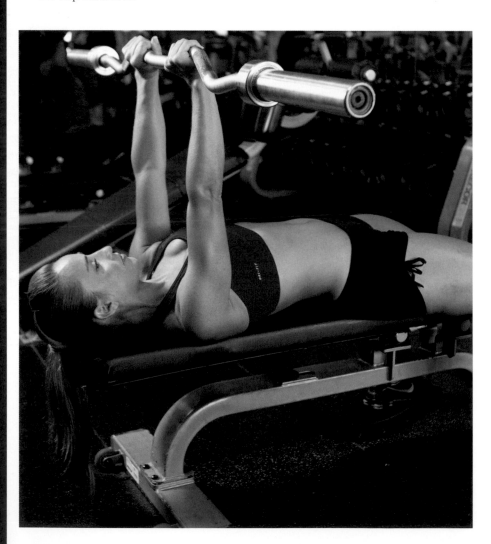

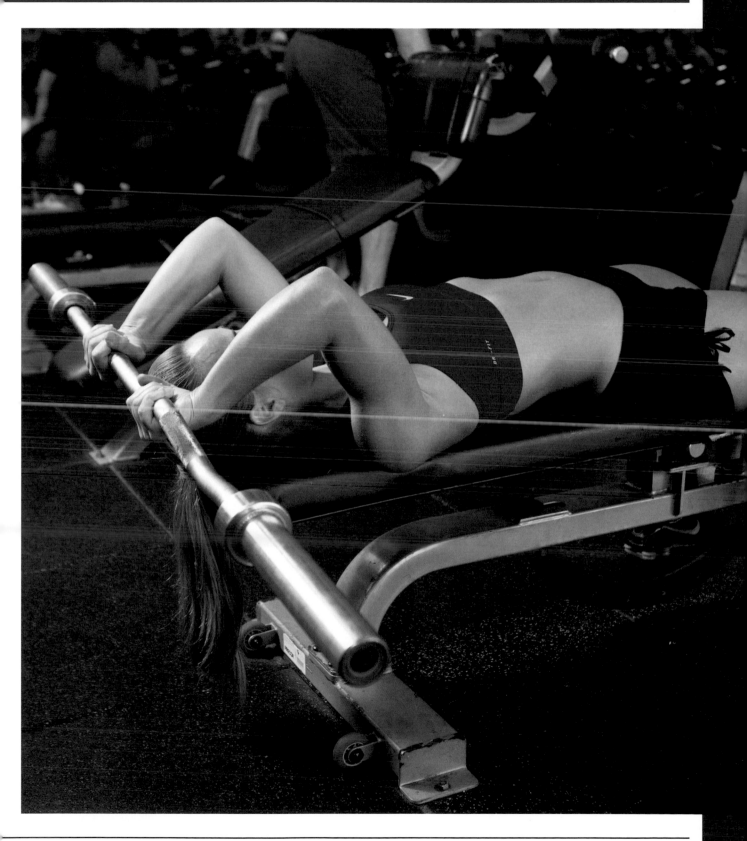

OVERHEAD DUMBBELL EXTENSION

PROGRESSION

1 Begin by sitting on a bench with a dumbbell pushed upward directly over your head with a clasped, palms-up grip placed against the inside of the top plate.

2 Start by bending your arms at the elbow behind your head while keeping your upper arms locked and the elbows in.

3 Raise your arms above your head to full lockout, and repeat for 10 to 12 repetitions.

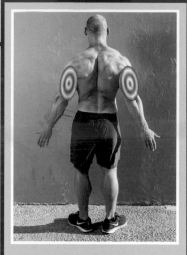

MUSCLE ACTION: PRIMARY ACTIVATION
- triceps brachii

ANCILLARY ACTIVATION
- rhomboideus
- erector spinae
- rectus abdominis

PROPER FORM
- Slow and controlled repetitions
- Keeping your upper arms braced and stabilized throughout the movement
- Keeping your elbows in

AVOID
- Excessive speed
- A short range of motion
- Flared elbows

BEGINNER MODIFICATION
- Try it with a lighter weight.

ADVANCED MODIFICATION
- Try it one arm at a time.

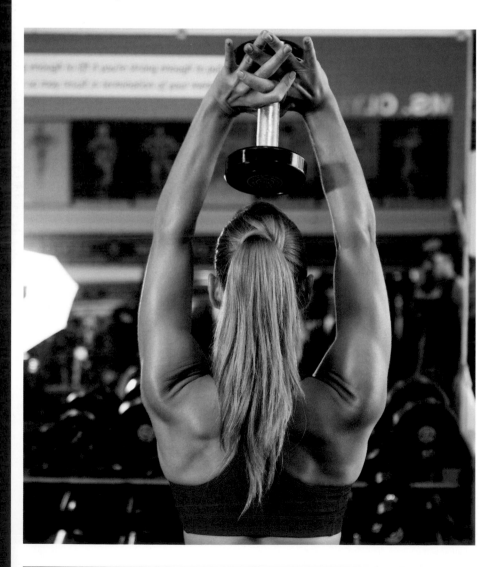

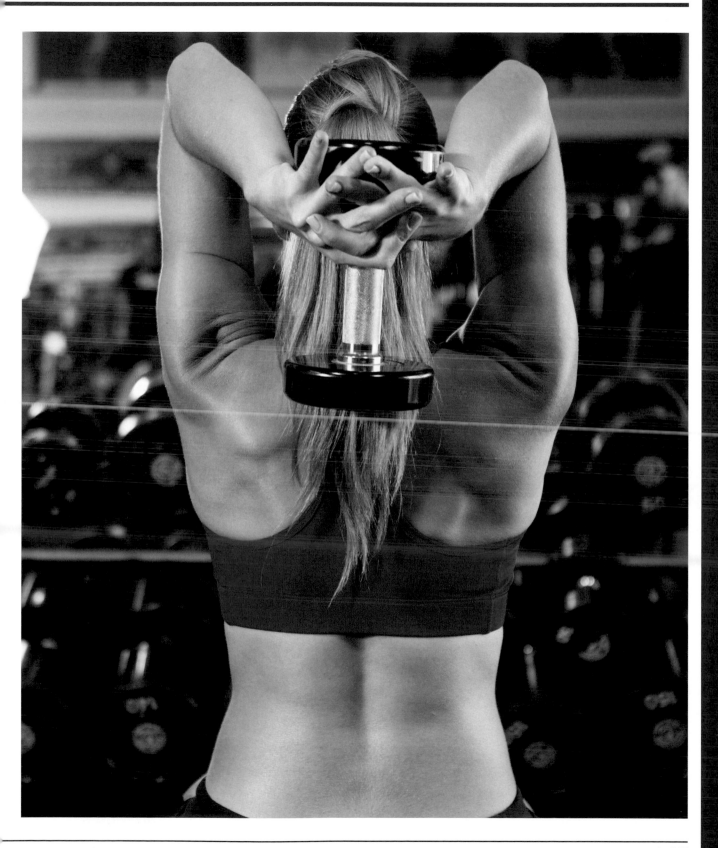

TRICEPS PUSHDOWN

PROGRESSION

1 Begin by standing in front of a cable stack with either a short bar or rope attached at the top pulley.

2 Take a close grip on the bar or rope, with your hands about 4 to 6 inches apart, and keep your elbows at your sides with your forearms parallel to the ground.

3 Push straight down until your arms are fully extended, and then slowly bend your arms back to the starting position, and repeat for 12 to 15 repetitions.

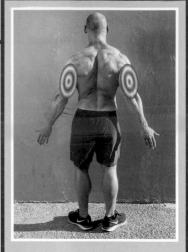

MUSCLE ACTION: PRIMARY ACTIVATION
- triceps brachii

ANCILLARY ACTIVATION
- rhomboideus
- erector spinae
- rectus abdominis

PROPER FORM
- Slow and controlled repetitions
- Keeping your elbows in at your sides
- A full and complete range of motion

AVOID
- Excessive speed
- A short range of motion
- Flaring your elbows out

BEGINNER MODIFICATION
- Try it with a lighter weight.

ADVANCED MODIFICATION
- Try it one arm at a time.

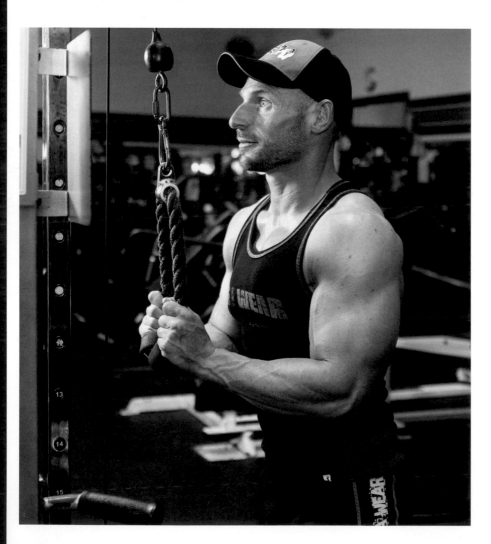

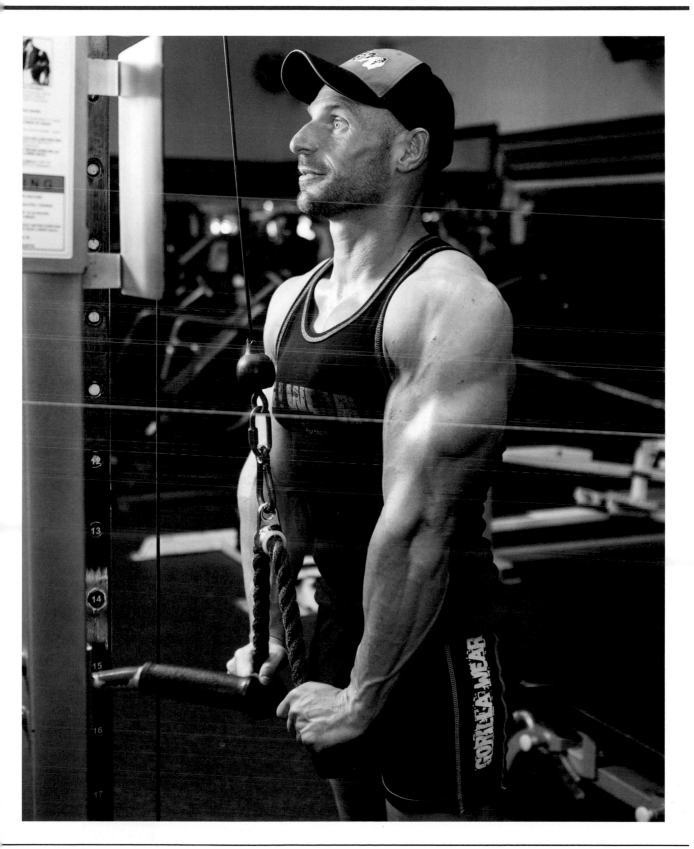

DUMBBELL KICKBACK

PROGRESSION

1 Begin in a standing position with a dumbbell in each hand and bend forward at the waist while keeping your upper arms at your sides and your back flat.

2 Extend your forearms back until your arms are fully extended and parallel to the ground.

3 Return to the starting position while moving only your forearms, and repeat for 12 to 15 repetitions.

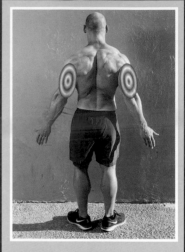

MUSCLE ACTION: PRIMARY ACTIVATION
- triceps brachii

ANCILLARY ACTIVATION
- erector spinae
- rectus abdominis

PROPER FORM
- Slow and controlled repetitions
- Keeping your elbows in
- Keeping your back flat

AVOID
- Excessive speed
- Dipping your upper arms below parallel to the ground
- A shortened range of motion

BEGINNER MODIFICATION
- Try it with a lighter weight.

ADVANCED MODIFICATION
- Try it with a rope attachment.

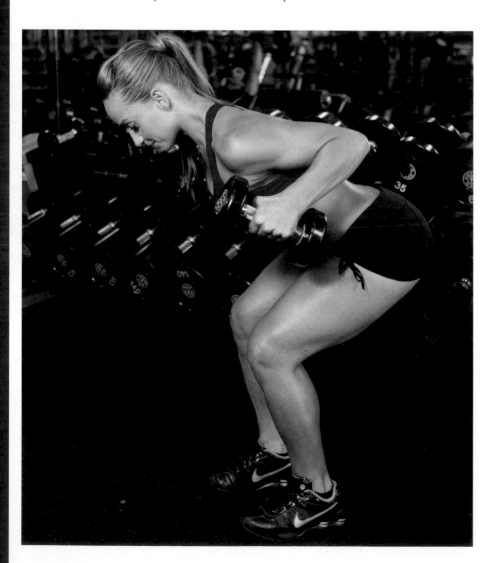

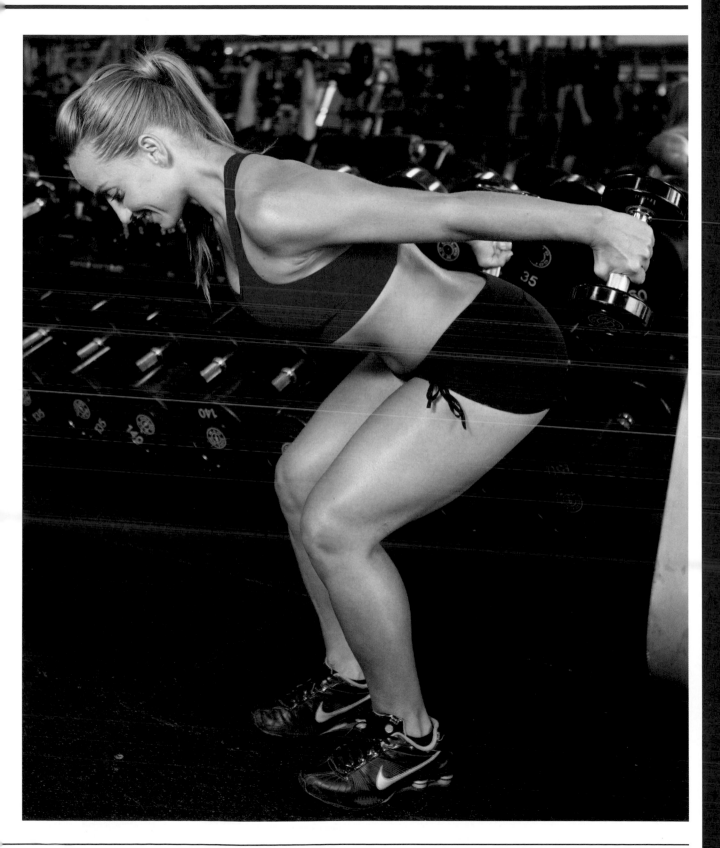

CRUNCH

PROGRESSION

1 Begin by lying down on your back with your legs bent and your palms placed on your ears with your elbows flared outward.

2 Raise your head and shoulders off the ground while contracting your trunk toward your pelvis, keeping your lower back grounded to the floor.

3 Lower and repeat for 25 repetitions.

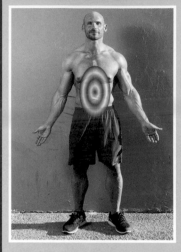

MUSCLE ACTION: PRIMARY ACTIVATION
- rectus abdominis

ANCILLARY ACTIVATION
- obliquus externus
- obliquus internus
- erector spinae

PROPER FORM
- Maintaining constant tension on the muscle
- Leading as if pulling from the belly button
- Contracting your abdominal muscles at the top

AVOID
- Using the neck
- Bouncy and speedy repetitions
- Raising your lower back off the ground

BEGINNER MODIFICATION
- Try it with straight legs.

ADVANCED MODIFICATION
- Try rotating your elbow toward its opposite knee as you come up.

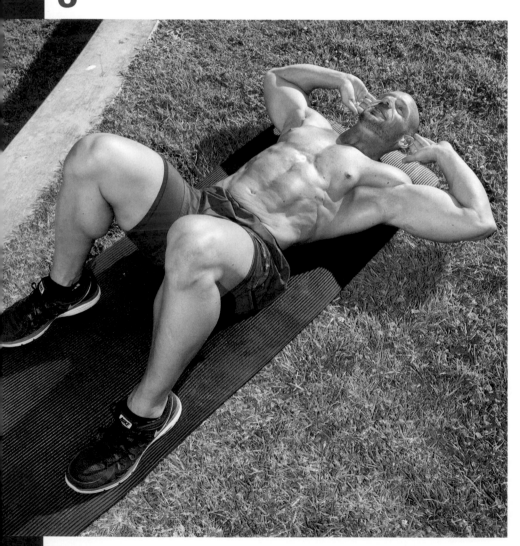

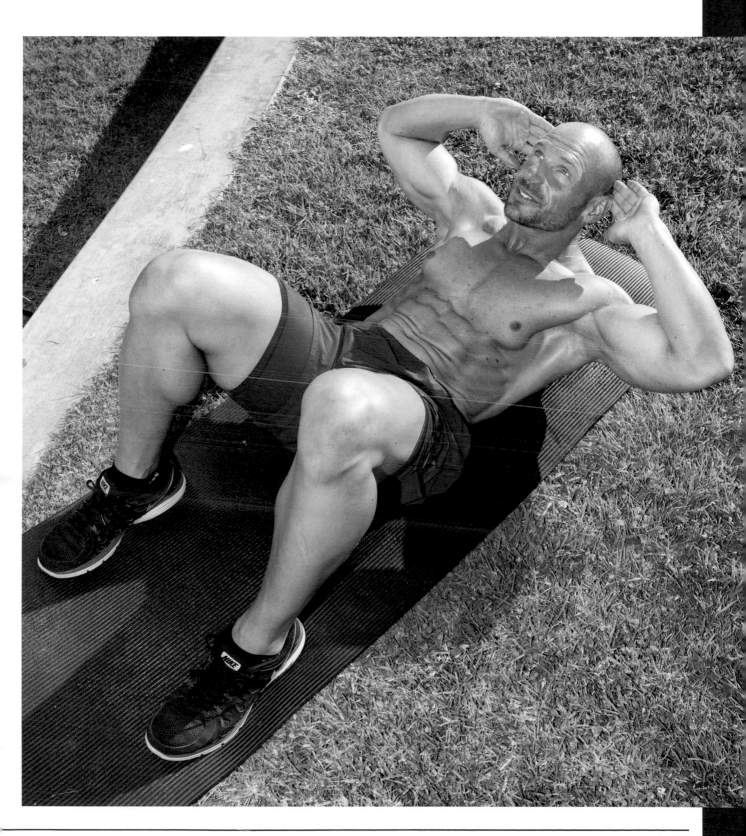

REVERSE CRUNCH

PROGRESSION

1 Begin by lying on your back on a flat bench with your arms behind your head, gripping the bench, and your legs bent to a 90-degree angle with your feet off the bench.

2 Roll your legs back into your midriff and lift your lower body a few inches off the bench.

3 Lower in a controlled manner while never allowing your feet to touch the bench, and repeat for 20 repetitions.

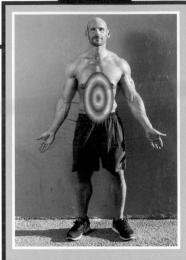

**MUSCLE ACTION:
PRIMARY ACTIVATION**
- rectus abdominis
- obliquus externus
- obliquus internus

ANCILLARY ACTIVATION
- erector spinae
- hip flexors

PROPER FORM
- A controlled range of motion
- A controlled return to the starting position
- Using your abdominals to lift your lower body

AVOID
- Excessive speed
- A shortened range of motion
- Using too much neck and/or lower back at the expense of your abdominals

BEGINNER MODIFICATION
- Try it with straight legs brought into your chest.

ADVANCED MODIFICATION
- Try it while holding a medicine ball between your upper thighs.

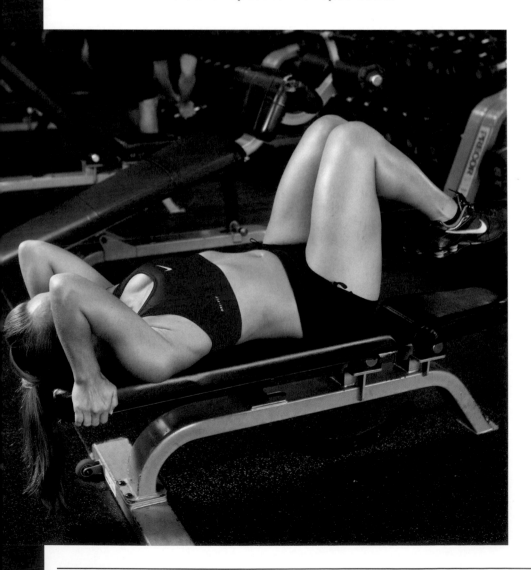

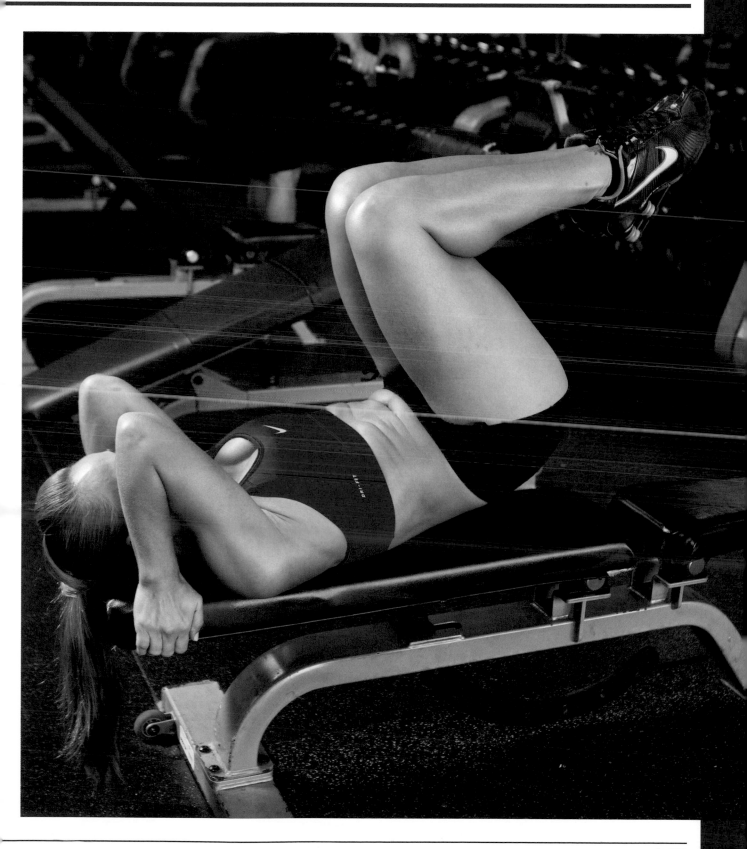

DOWN-UP

PROGRESSION

1 Begin in a facedown position supported on your forearms and toes.

2 Start by replacing one planted forearm with one hand and extend to the full lockout position.

3 Repeat with the other arm until in a completed push-up position, then reverse one arm at a time, going from planted hand to forearm, until back in the initial plank position for 15 complete repetitions.

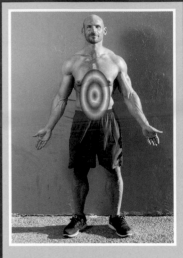

MUSCLE ACTION: PRIMARY ACTIVATION
- rectus abdominis
- erector spinae

ANCILLARY ACTIVATION
- gluteus maximus
- hip flexors
- triceps brachii
- pectoralis major
- tibialis anterior

PROPER FORM
- A controlled range of motion
- Keeping your body elevated parallel to the ground or slightly higher
- Primarily using your core to lift

AVOID
- Excessive speed
- Dipping your lower back below parallel to the ground
- Using too much neck and/or shoulders

BEGINNER MODIFICATION
- Try it on your knees.

ADVANCED MODIFICATION
- Try keeping one leg raised.

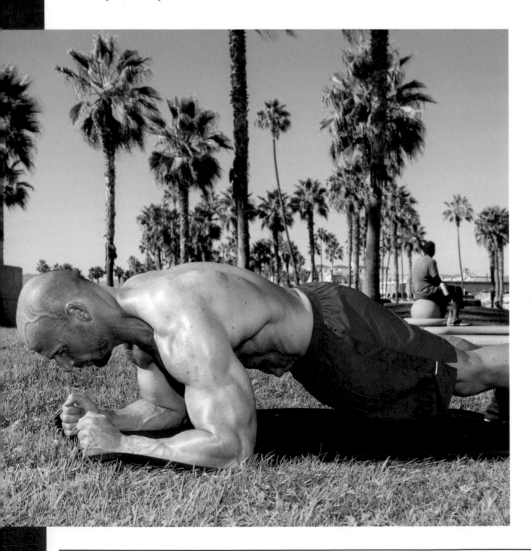

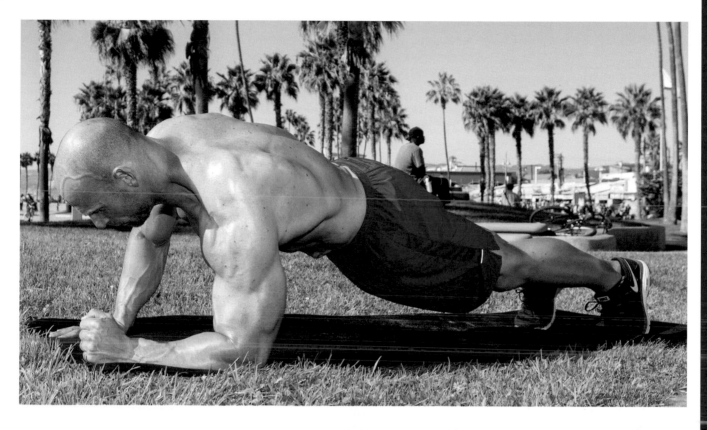

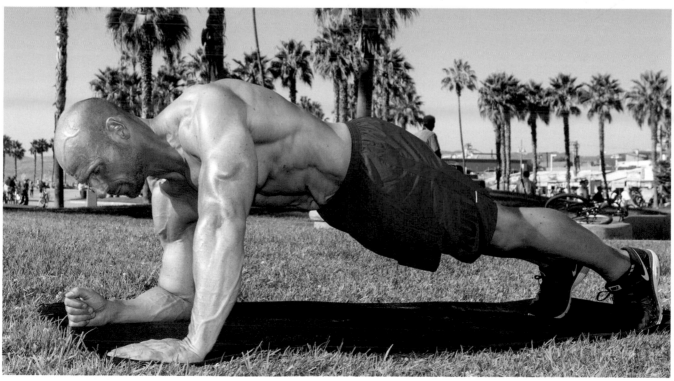

SEATED RUSSIAN TWIST

PROGRESSION

1 Begin in a seated position on the ground or an exercise mat, with your legs apart. Bend your legs slightly, flexing your feet upward to rest on your heels, as you hold your arms straight, hands together forming an arrow.

2 Lean back slightly to activate your core, and, while keeping a flat back, begin rotating from side to side for 20 complete and full rotations.

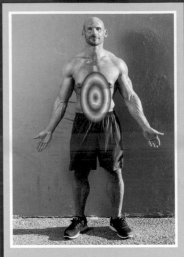

**MUSCLE ACTION:
PRIMARY ACTIVATION**
- rectus abdominis
- obliquus externus
- obliquus internus
- erector spinae

ANCILLARY ACTIVATION
- hip flexors

PROPER FORM
- Keeping a flat back throughout the movement
- Looking straight ahead
- Keeping your core engaged

AVOID
- Rounding your back
- Holding your breath
- Excessive speed

BEGINNER MODIFICATION
- Try completing one side's repetitions first before proceeding to the other side.

ADVANCED MODIFICATION
- Try it while holding a medicine ball.

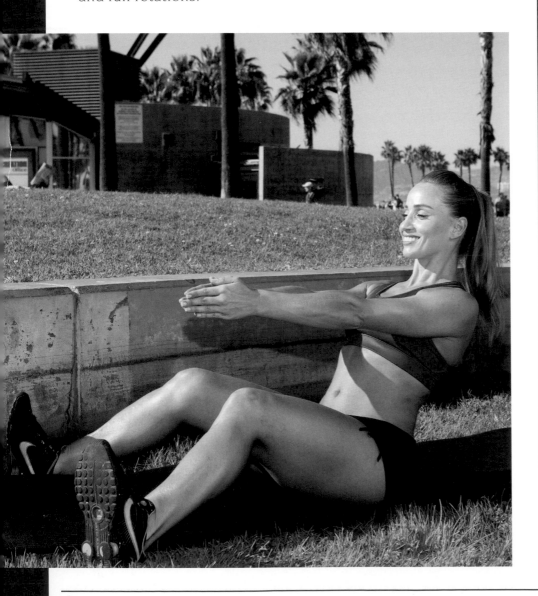

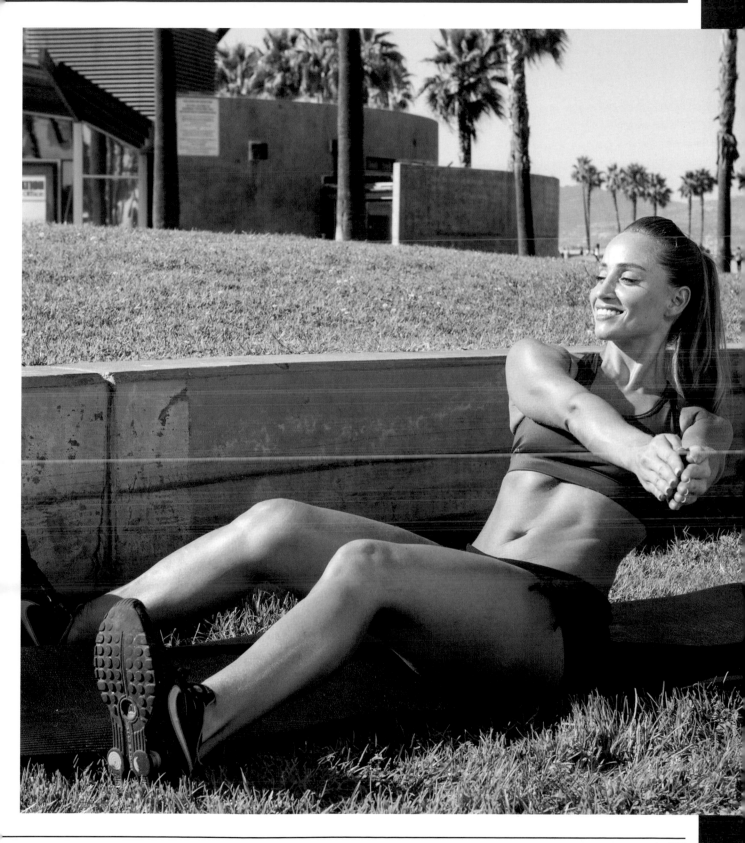

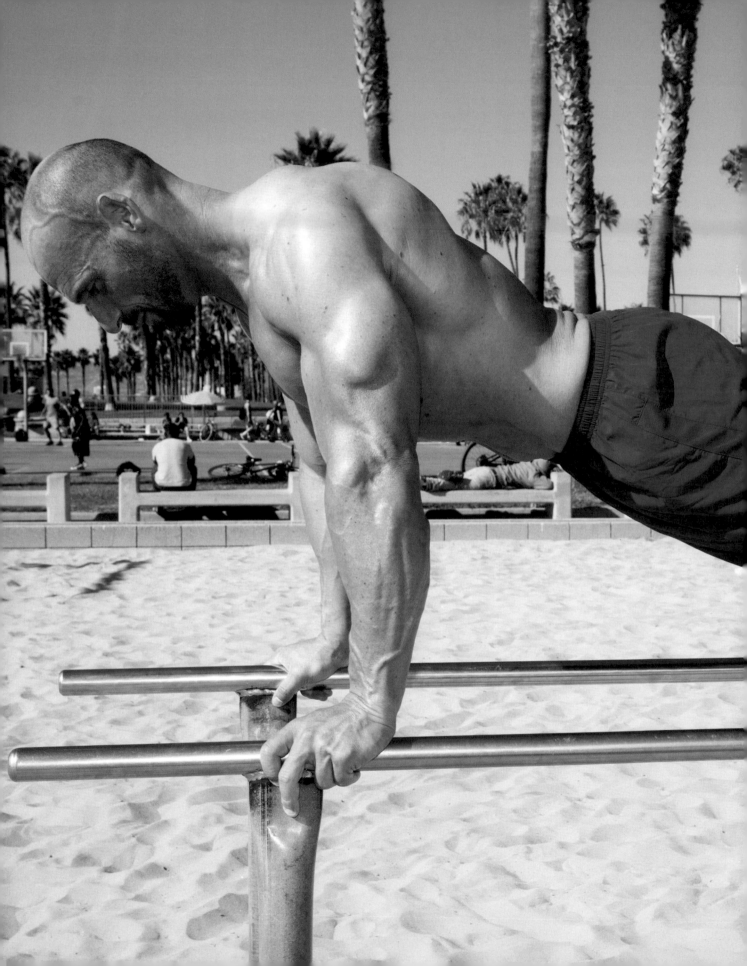

CHAPTER 6

THE OUTDOOR WORKOUT

Ideally, a gym workout is an important component of your Peak Physique program, but, of course, not everyone has access to a gym or even training equipment. Yet, if it worked for our ancestors, the outdoors will indeed work for you and your modern-day pursuit of a lean and strong body.

We all have access (sometimes limited due to climate) to the great outdoors. Parks, for example, make excellent substitutes for the sweaty indoors. In most of them, you can perform a near-infinite array of body-weight exercises. If your local park or recreational area also has some basic equipment, such as parallel bars, you can perform an even greater variety of exercises.

TAKE IT OUTSIDE

Whether you go to a park, your backyard or the seaside, don't be afraid to take a deep breath and head outside. The Outdoor Workout offers you unique benefits, such as quality time with Mother Nature and a fresh exercise perspective—both of which can be welcome breaks from the sometimes routine monotony of the gym.

In your pursuits toward physique excellence, use this full-body workout for a different type of stimulus—as well as greater cardiovascular expenditure—either as a break from your regular exercise routine or simply when the need and desire takes you.

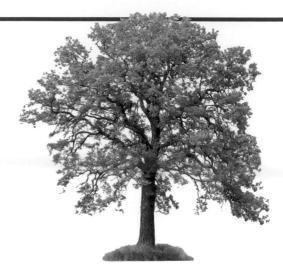

THE OUTDOOR WORKOUT

The Outdoor Workout is split into three circuits of exercises. Simply perform each exercise in the circuit back to back two times through, for the prescribed number of repetitions when on the go, and you'll not only stay on track, but further stimulate your body.

Circuit 1

Targets: Chest/Back/Arms
Exercises:

- Push-Up x 10–15
- Inverted Row x 10–12
- Vertical Dip x 8–10
- Superman x 15

Perform Circuit 1 twice and then proceed to Circuit 2.

Circuit 2

Targets: Glutes/Quadriceps/Hamstrings
Exercises:

- Sumo Squat x 15
- Forward Lunge x 12–15 per leg
- Bridge x 15–20
- Single-Leg Deadlift x 10 per leg

Perform Circuit 2 twice and then proceed to Circuit 3.

Circuit 3

Targets: Abdominals/Obliques/Spinal Extensors
Exercises:

- V-Up x 20
- Penguin Crunch x 10 per side
- Twisting Crunch x 20 per side
- Twisting Side Plank x 15 per side

Perform Circuit 3 twice, and you have concluded.

EXERCISE FOR TRAVELERS

What should you do if you are away from home and nowhere near your local gym?

For many of us, travel is a fact of life, whether for pleasure or business. For many of us, our livelihoods depend on our ability and willingness to get up and go when called upon. Yet, travel can put a serious strain on your peaking program. But with a little thought and planning, you will be able to successfully navigate both your nutrition and training protocol while away from home and continue to lose body fat and gain lean muscle tissue while logging in all those air miles.

PLAN AHEAD AND STAY MOTIVATED

The first step would be to look online when making your travel plans to see if your hotel is equipped with a gym. These days, most of the larger ones are, and you can usually find a plethora of resistance and cardiovascular equipment. And if while there the available equipment is foreign-looking to you, think of it as a great opportunity to try new angles and exercises.

While online, you may also want to look up the local eateries in your area and their menus, which as we've seen, almost always have a healthy choice. As far as packing for nutrition, although liquid is prohibited on planes, raw nuts, trail mix and protein powders are a go.

Additionally, a deflated Swiss ball, resistance bands and suspension kit are all portable exercise equipment that you can easily pack with your gym shorts and towel for keeping you fit on the go. You can even implement them privately in any hotel room. To further expedite your traveling program, you could conceivably call in a healthy food delivery to your hotel door and complete your workout while waiting for your meal following a long day of travel and work.

KEEPING FIT ANYWHERE

When traveling, you might not always have access to a hotel gym or a recreation park with stock equipment (and for those of you who do have access to outdoor equipment, sometimes less-than-receptive weather will not permit a workout of this kind). Furthermore, although bands and various resistance items can be deemed portable, sometimes luggage gets temporarily misplaced or lost. Add to this a hectic travel, sight-seeing or work day and your first instinct might be to jettison the workout entirely. To this I say nay!

To truly be deemed "portable," a workout needs to be a fail-safe plan that can be enacted nearly anywhere and anytime. To truly have you covered, a body-weight workout is the answer. Similar to the Outdoor Workout in structure and execution, the Portable Workout is a full-body workout that is short on content but high on stimulation, cardio, speed and efficacy.

THE PORTABLE WORKOUT

The Portable Workout is split into two circuits of exercises. Simply perform all the exercise in each circuit for the prescribed number of repetitions back to back three times through. Try keeping your rest between circuits down to 45 to 60 seconds (when able) for an increased challenge.

See the following pages for full exercise instructions.

Circuit 1
Exercises:

- Push-Up x 10–15
- Superman x 15
- Twisting Side Plank x 15 per side
- Sumo Squat x 15
- Forward Lunge x 12–15 per leg

Circuit 2
Exercises:

- Bridge x 15–20
- Single-Leg Deadlift x 10 per leg
- V-Up x 20
- Twisting Crunch x 20 per side
- Penguin Crunch x 10 per side

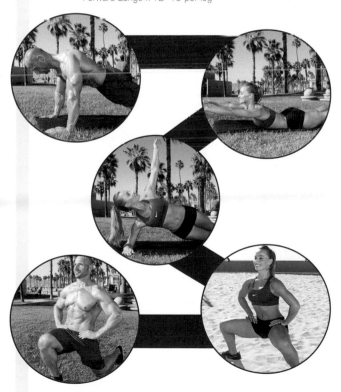

Perform Circuit 1 three times, and then rest for 45 to 60 seconds.

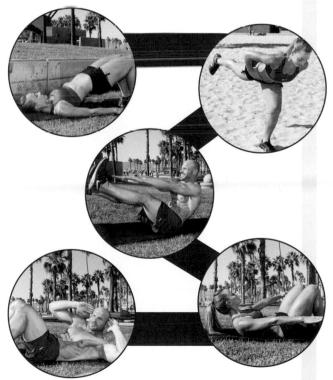

Perform Circuit 2 three times, and you have concluded.

PUSH-UP

PROGRESSION

1 Begin in a facedown position on your toes with your hands planted shoulder-width apart directly beneath your chest.

2 Start by lowering yourself until your upper arms are parallel to the ground, and then push your arms to full extension for 12 to 15 repetitions.

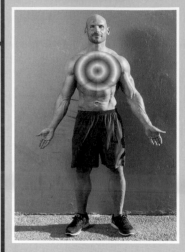

MUSCLE ACTION: PRIMARY ACTIVATION
- pectoralis major

ANCILLARY ACTIVATION
- deltoideus anterior
- triceps brachii
- rectus abdominis
- erector spinae
- rhomboideus

PROPER FORM
- Slow and controlled repetitions
- Keeping your torso stabilized and your upper body straight
- Engaging your core

AVOID
- Excessive speed
- Shallow or bouncy repetitions
- Allowing your lower back to dip down too far

BEGINNER MODIFICATION
- Try it on your knees.

ADVANCED MODIFICATION
- Try it with one leg raised.

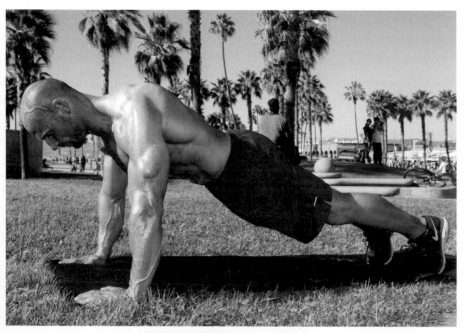

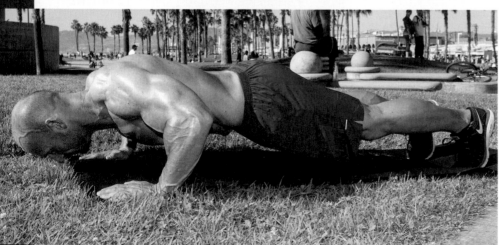

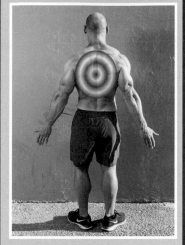

**MUSCLE ACTION:
PRIMARY ACTIVATION**

- latissimus dorsi

ANCILLARY ACTIVATION

- biceps brachii
- trapezius
- rhomboideus
- forearm extensors
- forearm flexors

PROPER FORM

- A controlled return to the starting position
- Pulling your elbows down and back
- Contracting each repetition at the top of the movement

AVOID

- Bending your wrists
- Excessive body swinging
- Using your biceps excessively instead of your back

BEGINNER MODIFICATION

- Try it with bent knees.

ADVANCED MODIFICATION

- Try it with additional resistance held between your thighs.

INVERTED ROW

PROGRESSION

1 Begin by hanging below a bar at arms' length with an overhand, shoulder-width grip and your legs straight out in front of you while supported on your heels.

2 Start by pulling your body toward the bar until your nipple line is nearly touching the bar, while drawing your shoulder blades back.

3 Lower back to the starting position and repeat for 10 to 12 repetitions.

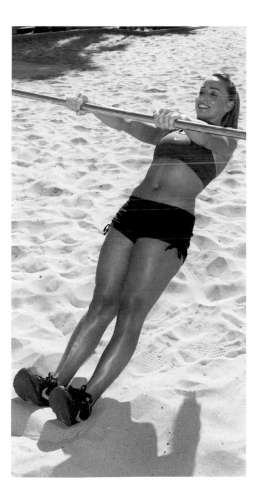

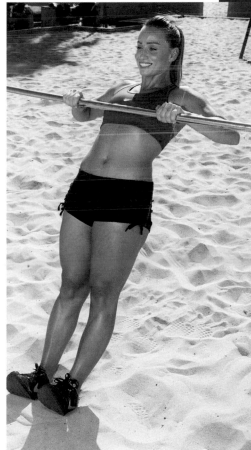

VERTICAL DIP

PROGRESSION

1 Begin by standing between a pair of dip bars with your hands placed firmly on the bars. Bend your knees and cross your legs at the ankles, lowering yourself until your upper arms are parallel to the ground.

2 Push yourself up to lockout and repeat the movement for 8 to 10 full repetitions.

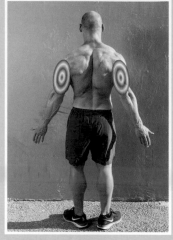

**MUSCLE ACTION:
PRIMARY ACTIVATION**
• triceps brachii

ANCILLARY ACTIVATION
• deltoideus anterior
• pectoralis major
• rectus abdominis
• rhomboideus

PROPER FORM
• A controlled lowering
• A stabilized torso and an upright upper body
• A full range of motion

AVOID
• Excessive speed
• Shallow or bouncy repetitions
• Leaning too far forward

BEGINNER MODIFICATION
• Have someone assist you by holding you at your feet

ADVANCED MODIFICATION
• Try it with additional resistance held between your feet.

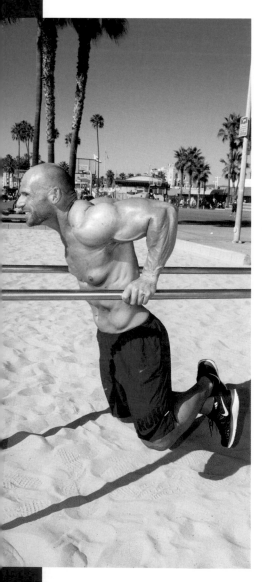

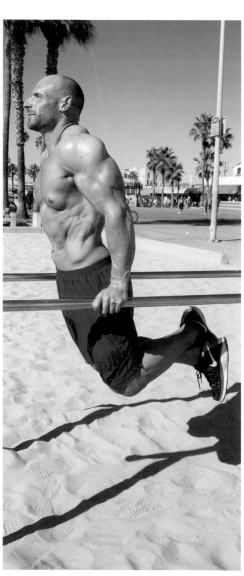

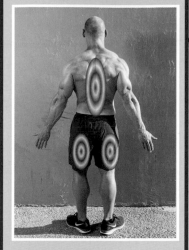

MUSCLE ACTION:
PRIMARY ACTIVATION

- erector spinae
- gluteus maximus

ANCILLARY ACTIVATION

- rectus abdominis
- hip flexors
- deltoideus anterior
- deltoideus medialis
- deltoideus posterior
- hamstrings

PROPER FORM
- A controlled range of motion
- Long legs and arms
- Primarily lifting with your lower back

AVOID
- Excessive speed
- A shortened range of motion
- Using too much neck

BEGINNER MODIFICATION
- Try raising just your arms.

ADVANCED MODIFICATION
- Try it holding a light pair of dumbbells.

SUPERMAN

PROGRESSION

1 Begin by lying facedown with your arms and legs fully lengthened and stretched out.

2 Raise both arms and legs simultaneously, while squeezing the glutes at the top portion, and then lowering for 15 repetitions.

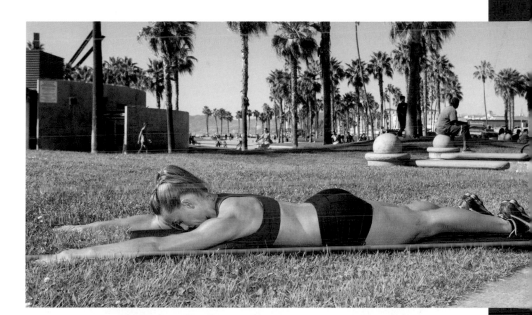

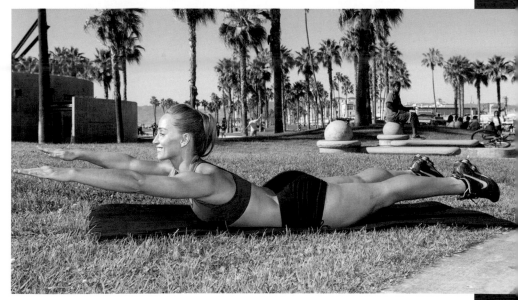

SUMO SQUAT

PROGRESSION

1 Begin standing with your feet spaced well beyond shoulder-width apart and your toes pointed slightly outward.

2 Stick your rear out as you bend at the knees, while keeping your back flat and lowering yourself toward the ground until your thighs are parallel to it.

3 Push through your heels to stand tall, and repeat the full movement for 15 repetitions.

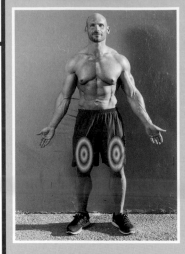

**MUSCLE ACTION:
PRIMARY ACTIVATION**
- inner thighs
- quadriceps femoris
- gluteus maximus
- hamstrings

ANCILLARY ACTIVATION
- erector spinae
- transversus abdominis
- hip abductors
- hip adductors
- soleus
- gastrocnemius

PROPER FORM
- Squatting until your thighs are parallel to the ground
- A controlled descent
- Pushing through your heels to drive the movement

AVOID
- Hyperextending your knees past your feet
- A rounded back
- A shortened range of motion

BEGINNER MODIFICATION
- Try it braced against a wall

ADVANCED MODIFICATION
- A closer stance will increase the range of motion

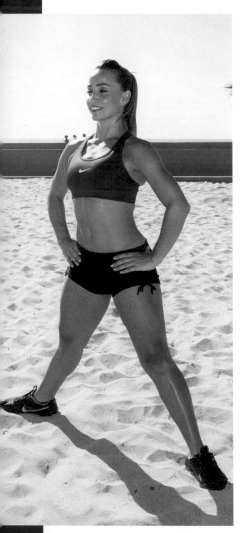

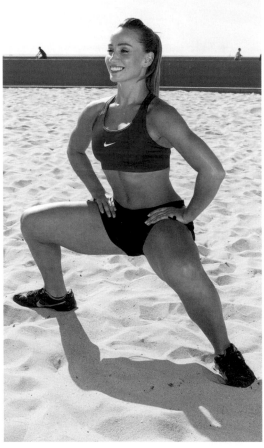

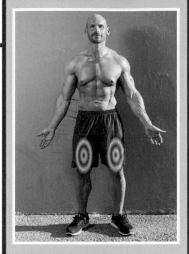

MUSCLE ACTION:
PRIMARY ACTIVATION
- quadriceps femoris
- gluteus maximus
- hamstrings

ANCILLARY ACTIVATION
- erector spinae
- transversus abdominis
- hip abductors
- hip adductors
- soleus
- gastrocnemius

PROPER FORM
- Pushing through the front heel to drive the movement
- Lunging until your front thigh is parallel to the ground
- Allowing the rear heel to rise

AVOID
- Allowing the knee to hyper-extend past the front foot
- Keeping the rear heel flat
- A slouched posture

BEGINNER MODIFICATION
- Try it holding a pole in hand for support.

ADVANCED MODIFICATION
- Try it with a barbell across your rear shoulders.

FORWARD LUNGE

PROGRESSION

1 Begin in a standing position with your hands resting on your hips and start by taking one giant step forward with one leg.

2 Bend both legs until your front thigh is parallel to the ground and your back heel is up.

3 Push through your front heel as you return your front leg back to the starting position, and then repeat for 12 to 15 repetitions per leg.

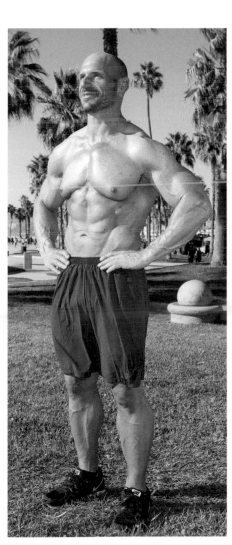
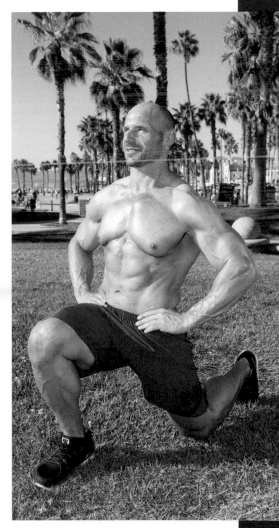

BRIDGE

PROGRESSION

1 Begin by lying on your back with your legs bent and your feet flat on the ground.

2 Push your heels into the ground, while raising your pelvis up until you're bridged at the top.

3 Squeeze your glutes at the top, and then lower and repeat for 15 to 20 repetitions.

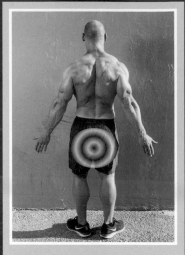

MUSCLE ACTION: PRIMARY ACTIVATION
- gluteus maximus
- hamstrings

ANCILLARY ACTIVATION
- erector spinae
- rectus abdominis

PROPER FORM
- A controlled range of motion
- Bent legs throughout
- Pushing through your heels

AVOID
- Speedy repetitions
- Lengthening your legs
- A shortened range of motion

BEGINNER MODIFICATION
- Try performing fewer but perfect repetitions per set.

ADVANCED MODIFICATION
- Try lifting one leg while in the bridge position.

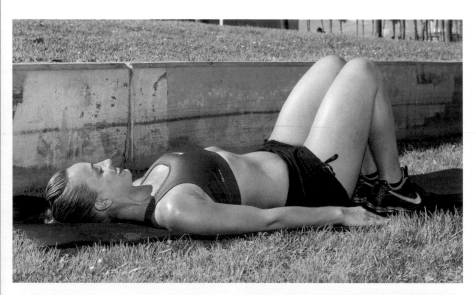

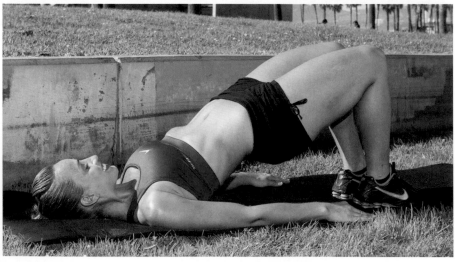

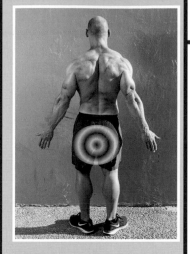

MUSCLE ACTION:
PRIMARY ACTIVATION
- gluteus maximus
- hamstrings

ANCILLARY ACTIVATION
- erector spinae
- rectus abdominis

PROPER FORM
- Maintaining a flat back
- Keeping your planted leg straight
- A controlled and full range of motion

AVOID
- Rounding your back
- Imbalance
- Not keeping your back leg in sync with your torso

BEGINNER MODIFICATION
- Try it holding a pole in hand for support.

ADVANCED MODIFICATION
- Try it with a light barbell or pair of dumbbells.

SINGLE-LEG DEADLIFT

PROGRESSION

1 Begin in a standing position with the majority of your weight placed on one heel while keeping the other foot very soft to the ground, just barely touching it.

2 Start by bending forward at the waist while simultaneously lifting your soft leg until both your leg and back are near parallel to the ground and your hands remain on your hips.

3 Return to the starting position 10 times, and then switch legs. Repeat 10 times on the other leg, for a total of 20 repetitions.

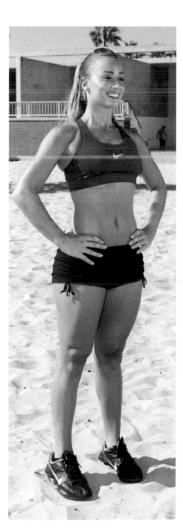

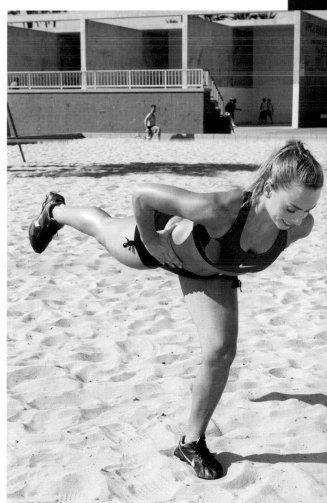

V-UP

PROGRESSION

1 Begin by lying flat on your back with your arms and legs elongated and your lower back firmly against the ground.

2 Simultaneously raise both your arms and legs toward one another so that your arms are nearly touching your feet while maintaining a flat back. Lower and repeat for 20 repetitions.

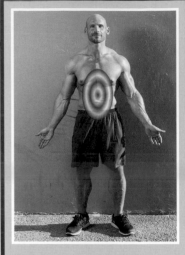

**MUSCLE ACTION:
PRIMARY ACTIVATION**
- rectus abdominis
- erector spinae

ANCILLARY ACTIVATION
- deltoideus anterior
- deltoideus medialis
- deltoideus posterior
- hip flexors
- quadriceps femoris
- gluteus maximus
- hamstrings

PROPER FORM
- Lengthened arms and legs
- A linear motion
- Your lower back flat against the ground

AVOID
- A haphazard pattern
- Excessive speed or swinging
- Not keeping your torso straight on

BEGINNER MODIFICATION
- Try a shorter range of motion.

ADVANCED MODIFICATION
- Try it with ankle weights.

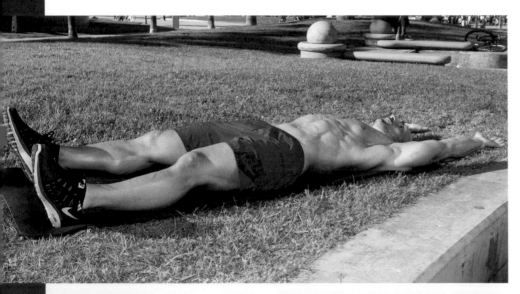

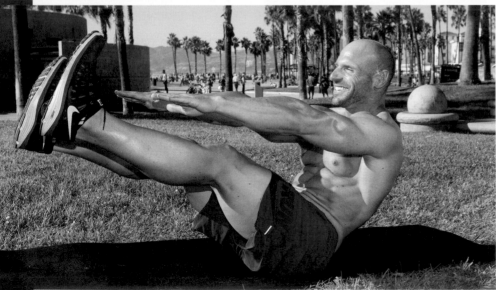

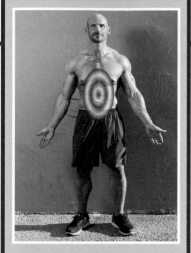

**MUSCLE ACTION:
PRIMARY ACTIVATION**
- rectus abdominis
- obliquus externus
- obliquus internus

ANCILLARY ACTIVATION
- erector spinae

PROPER FORM
- Leading from your belly button
- Short and precise reaching motions
- Keeping your lower back pressed against the ground

AVOID
- Using your neck
- Too much forward motion
- Holding your breath

BEGINNER MODIFICATION
- Try it one side at a time.

ADVANCED MODIFICATION
- Try it with wrist weights.

PENGUIN CRUNCH

PROGRESSION

1 Begin on your back with your head elevated, your legs bent and your arms at your sides while slightly elevated off the ground.

2 Move your arms both forward and upward, alternately, toward their respective sides.

3 Lower and repeat 20 repetitions per side.

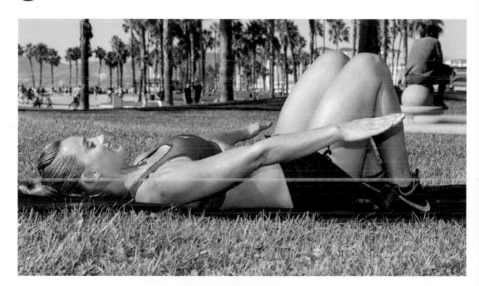

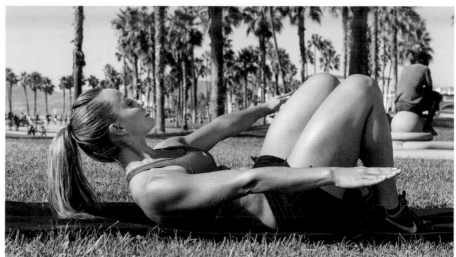

TWISTING CRUNCH

PROGRESSION

1 Begin lying down on your back with your legs bent and your palms placed on your ears with your elbows flared outward.

2 Raise your head and shoulders off the ground while contracting your trunk toward your waist as you rotate your elbow toward its opposite knee, then, lower and repeat with the other side for 20 repetitions per side.

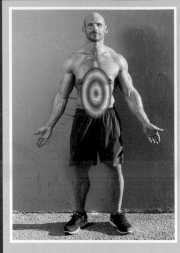

MUSCLE ACTION: PRIMARY ACTIVATION
- rectus abdominis
- obliquus externus
- obliquus internus

ANCILLARY ACTIVATION
- erector spinae

PROPER FORM
- Maintaining constant tension on the muscle
- Leading as if pulling from the belly button
- Contracting the muscles at the top

AVOID
- Using the neck
- Bouncy and speedy repetitions
- Raising your lower back off the ground

BEGINNER MODIFICATION
- Try a shorter range of motion.

ADVANCED MODIFICATION
- Try it holding a light pair of dumbbells.

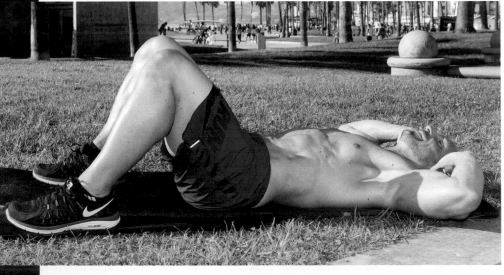

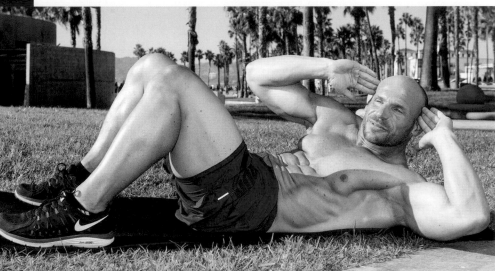

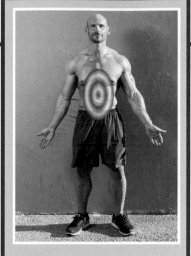

MUSCLE ACTION:
PRIMARY ACTIVATION
- transversus abdominis
- erector spinae
- obliques

ANCILLARY ACTIVATION
- triceps brachii
- deltoideus anterior
- deltoideus medialis
- deltoideus posterior
- hip flexors
- hip extensors
- gluteus maximus
- hamstrings

PROPER FORM
- Keeping your body elevated
- Steadily breathing throughout the exercise
- Keeping your abdominals contracted

AVOID
- Overly rotating your body
- Crashing back to the ground
- Using too much shoulders and upper back

BEGINNER MODIFICATION
- Try it without the rotation.

ADVANCED MODIFICATION
- Try it with one leg elevated.

TWISTING SIDE PLANK
PROGRESSION

1 Begin by lying on your side with your legs straight and parallel to each other.

2 Bend your bottom arm to a 90-degree angle with your knuckles facing forward as you push off your forearm while raising your hips off the ground until your body is in one straight line.

3 With your free hand, reach under your abdomen while simultaneously twisting your hips forward and then backward as you reach the outstretched arm above you. Perform 15 repetitions per side.

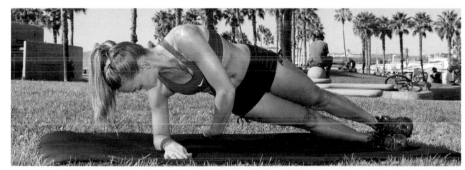

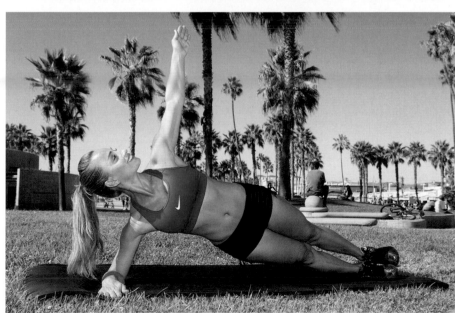

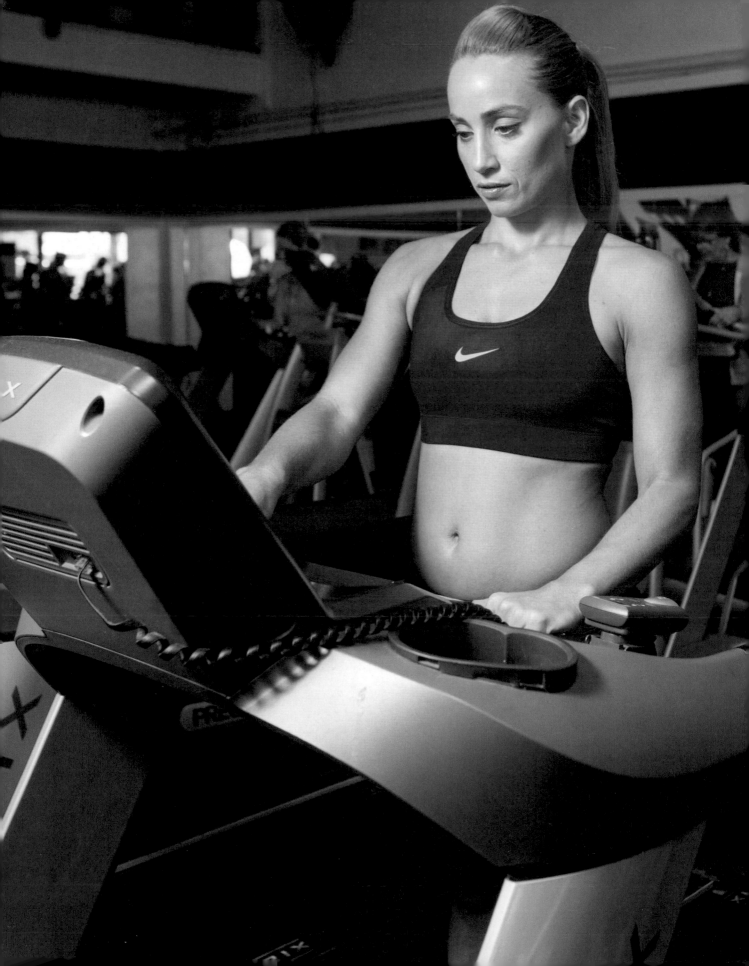

CHAPTER 7

CARDIO, COOL-DOWNS AND OTHER CONSIDERATIONS

The subject of cardio was covered briefly in chapter 2, but its role in your program is not to be minimized and requires further explanation. I even wanted to place this chapter prior to the actual exercise chapters but to maintain the integrity of the workouts themselves—that is resistance training performed first, followed by cardio—I felt its placement here well justified.

So we know that cardio is not only performed for the heart and lungs, but also because it helps rid the body of stored adipose (fat). We also know that aside from a light 5-to-10-minute warm-up, cardio should be done after resistance training to prevent fatigue and burnout during the workout. We should also know that cardio starts to burn fat as fuel roughly 20 minutes in.

It is my experience that cardio performed for more than 45 minutes can cut into muscle tissue, affect recovery and make you ravenous following its completion. And for those of you who typically perform an hour or more of cardio daily and swear by it, omitting resistance training in the process, is your body currently firm, or is it mushy to the touch? And are you famished come dinner time, or satiated? Cardio: 30 to 40 minutes is optimal.

TIMING IS EVERYTHING

It is important to never eat right before cardio activity, for you'll simply burn what you just ate rather than speed up your metabolism. It boggles my mind when I see someone drinking an energy drink or eating a protein bar while performing cardio. And I'm not talking about a warm-up. I'm talking about an intense full-blown cardio session. To me this is like running the car heater and air conditioner at the same time (if that were possible). Cardio's proper placement is either directly following resistance training or first thing in the morning on an empty stomach.

I am not concerned with how many calories I burn during cardio—those calories are replaced at my next meal. I am concerned with speeding up my metabolism, the rate at which stored fat is utilized by the body. To accomplish this, stay within the target fat-burning zone. You can easily find this zone by taking your age and subtracting it from the number 220. This is your maximum heart rate, and by multiplying it from .65 to .85, you can find the zone in which you should remain for optimal fat burning. As an example, a 40-year-old man's maximum heart rate is 180. For fat burning purposes, he wants to stay within 117 to 153 beats per minute. As an additional rule of thumb, when performing cardio, if you are out of breath and can't hold a conversation, the intensity is too high, and you may risk burning muscle tissue.

WATCHING YOUR PROGRESS

Our plan here calls for a minimum of three 30-minute cardio sessions per week. As the weeks progress, that number will climb to as high as five 40-minute sessions per week. This coupled with the three-to-four day resistance split routine and five clean meals per day will radically change your physique from week 1 to week 12. Again, it's not so much about doing more, it's about doing it better and doing it consistently.

It's also about keeping weekly updated pictures of your body, preferably taken from all four sides that are, if you like, for your eyes only. Compare the just-taken photos with those of the week before and you will see definite progress as you ascend through the program. When I was competing, every week I would take video footage of my body from all angles. It was always amusing and brought a big smile to my face when fast-forwarding and seeing all that fat seemingly melt off to reveal the lean musculature underneath. If it were only that easy. Is it easy? No. Is it attainable? Yes, 100 percent, yes!

It is crucial to never work outside your comfort zone. If it feels too intense, it most probably is. Someone who has not worked out in a long time is not going to do very well if placed on an incline treadmill and told to run or even walk at a brisk pace. It is not important how strong you are or how quickly you are able to complete a given workout. What matters is that you lay down a brick per day. As the bricks and days pile up, one day, you will have erected a solid foundation and eventually a full house.

ON STRETCHING

Stretching is important to help remove toxins (lactic acid) from the body following your workout, increase your range of motion, reduce muscle soreness and to help transport nutrients more efficiently to areas of fatigue, all in an effort to quicken the repair process. A common misconception says to stretch prior to exercise, but that is tantamount to pulling on a frozen chicken, which could result in muscle tears. The body responds best to stretching both during and after exercise, when it is hot and malleable. If you still insist on stretching prior to exercise, however, you could conceivably stretch safely following some light cycling or warm-up.

You can include the following stretches in your training program, depending on the training day. They are individually labeled by body part. Simply perform each stretch as called for, holding each for 15 to 30 seconds at the conclusion of your resistance training and prior to your cardiovascular work.

Chest Stretch

Begin in a standing position with your arms drawn behind you with your elbows straight, your fingers interlocked and your palms facing downward. Extend your arms away from you while squeezing your shoulder blades together and keeping your abdominals tensed.

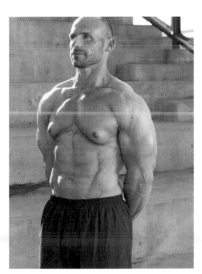

Upper Back

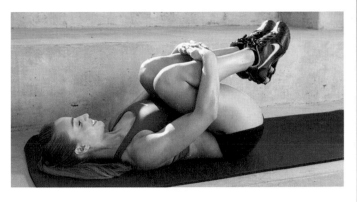

Begin standing in front of a pole with one arm outstretched, gripping the pole with your palm facing away from you. Lean both back and toward the side your palm is facing, feeling a deep stretch in your latissimus dorsi. Hold, and then switch sides.

Lower Back

Begin lying on your back with your legs bent and your fingers interlocked around your shins while you pull your legs into your chest.

Quadriceps

Begin in a standing position with one leg bent and your same-sided hand holding onto your toes. Lean forward while maintaining a flat back, feeling a tremendous stretch in your quadriceps.

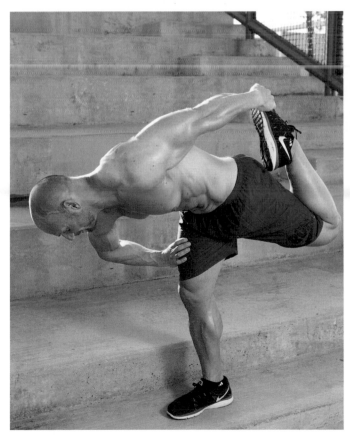

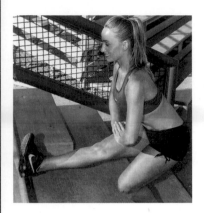

Hamstrings

Begin in a standing position with one leg stretched in front of you on a surface preferably higher than your navel. Keeping that leg straight and your other foot planted on the ground, lean backward feeling an intense stretch in your hamstrings.

Calves

Begin in a standing position facing a wall with one leg bent and that foot touching the wall and the other leg behind you, straight and with your heel flat on the ground. Hold, and then switch legs.

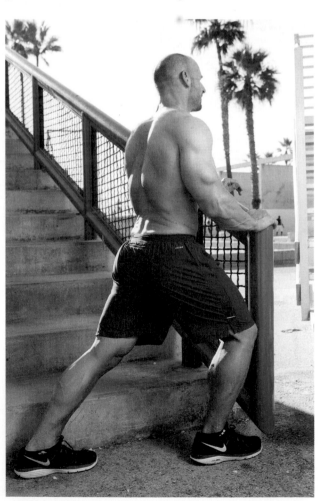

Shoulders

Begin seated or standing with one arm drawn across the front of your chest while holding that elbow with your opposite hand. Pull the stretched arm across the front of your body while keeping your shoulders down. Hold, and then switch arms.

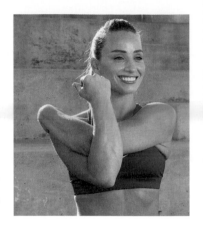

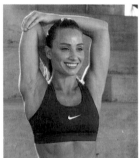

Triceps

Begin seated or standing with one arm above your head and bent at the elbow while holding that elbow with your opposite hand. Pull the stretched arm across the back of your head while keeping your upper arm locked. Hold, and then switch arms.

Biceps

Begin in a standing position with one arm outstretched to your side and that palm placed against a pole. Turn your upper body in toward the pole, hold, and then switch arms.

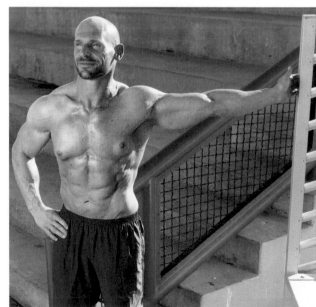

ON BREATHING

At the beginning of a set, clients often ask me, "How do I breathe?" My reply is always, "naturally," before I go further into detail. While it is true to keep breathing naturally, it is even more important to just keep breathing. Holding your breath during exercise (which for many is the norm for whatever the reason) can actually prove fatal. Some feel holding the breath will allow for a more explosive lift or increased focus or performance, but it could also lead to your last. Quite simply, inhale on the negative or stretch portion of a repetition (performed slowly), such as the descent during a squat. You'll want to exhale on the positive or contracted portion of the repetition (performed explosively), such as the ascent during a squat. Inhale on the lowering of the bar during a bench press, and exhale as you push it back up to full lockout.

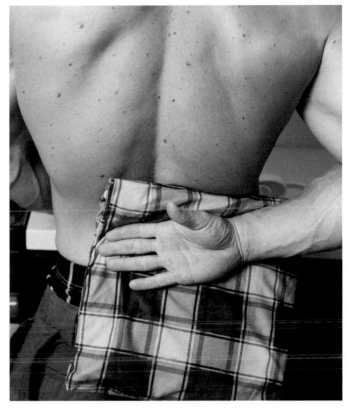

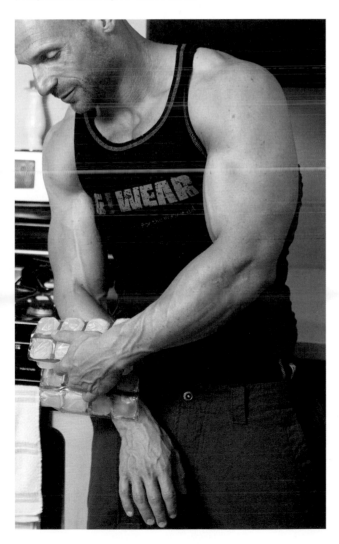

ON INJURY

In the movie *The Program*, James Caan plays a collegiate football coach and can be seen mouthing to a fallen player "Are you injured or are you hurt? If you're hurt you can still play, if you're injured you can't."

Oftentimes injuries begin outside of the gym, or as phrased earlier, the hammer is cocked outside the gym and the bullet fired in it. Aside from warming up and stretching, it is important to never rush your workout and stay attuned to your body. Listen to it. If a movement or posture doesn't feel right, switch to something else. Often a different angle or even grip can change a potentially painful movement into one you can perform pain-free. Be instinctive. If something feels off or amiss, leave the battle zone and return the next day, when you will most probably be feeling better.

In the eternal Ice versus Heat debate, it is important to know when and why to use which. Use ice to reduce swelling, pain and inflammation, such as during a sprain. Use heat when there is no inflammation or swelling in an effort to make tissue malleable such as a stiff lower back. It is also important to not stretch a muscle that is in pain or possibly injured.

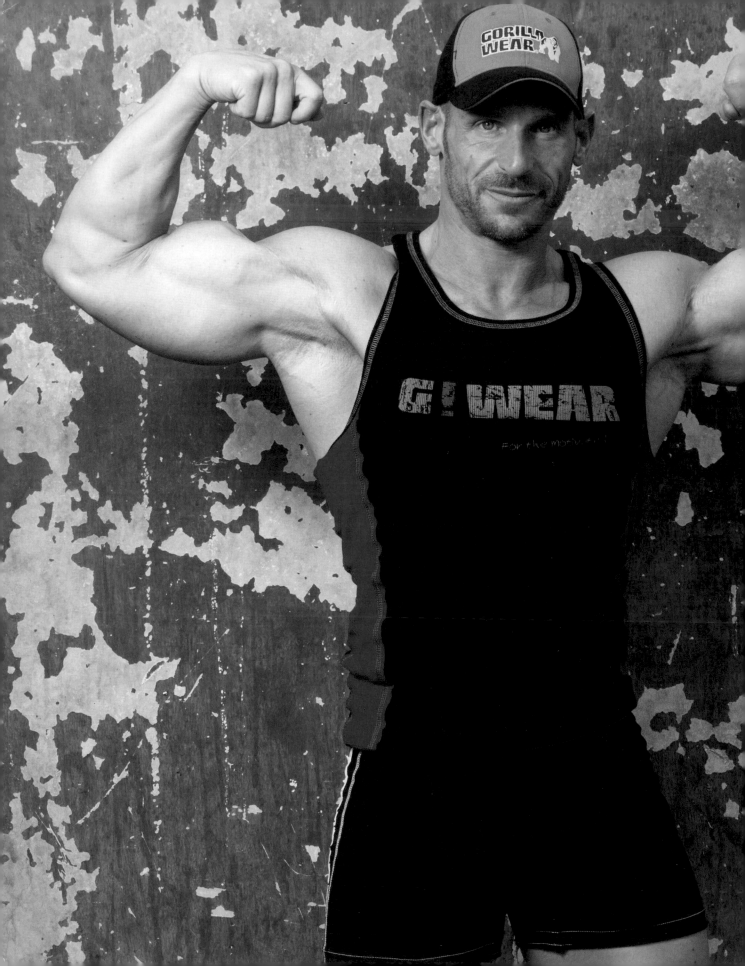

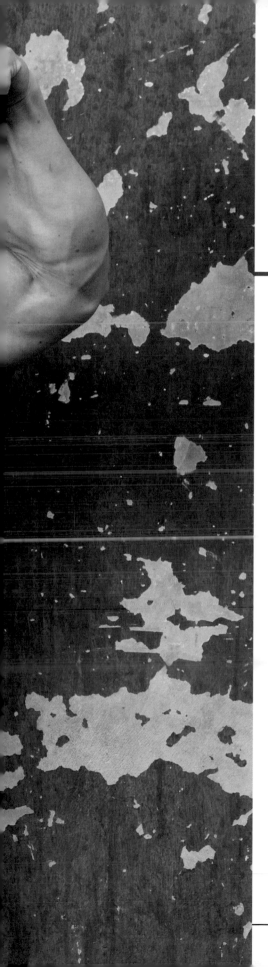

CHAPTER 8

REMOTIVATION

Sure, I've already discussed motivation way back in chapter 3, but one thing I've learned over the years is that defining and beginning a goal or process is nowhere near the most difficult part of a journey. At the onset it's quite exciting and fun to be fueled and driven toward bettering yourself. It's at a point later in the journey, when the day-to-day grind and slow accumulation of gains turns into plateaus or even abysses that you'll need motivation more than ever.

TAKE THE LEAD

Why does this pattern emerge? Sometimes you might feel that you're not seeing results fast enough, or maybe a friend or colleague chimes in with an opinion on what you might be doing "wrong." Doubts and negativity can creep up in your mind, leading to behavior-altering missteps. Life itself certainly doesn't slow down or move over to allow you ample time for your physique endeavors. Whatever the case, though, I want you to stop doubting right now. I want you to remember what brought you to this point in the first place. I want you to remember the stakes and what you have sacrificed to come this far. Again, begin to get your body in order by taking the lead with your mind.

MY OWN JOURNEY

My own peaking journey began on June 17, 2013, when I was 120 pounds lighter and yet 35 pounds heavier. You see, my fiancée left, and I had indulged in far too many cheat meals. I decided then to leave the self-sabotaging behavior behind and begin a journey back to me.

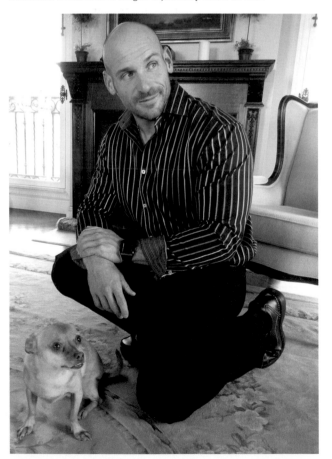

What you see on these pages is me today. Throughout my journey, I kept on track because I was hell-bent on bringing to the world my template for reclaiming you. But before doing so, I had to reclaim myself. So I set up a photo shoot, assembled new and flattering clothes (that would only fit if I got back into top shape), listened to a lot of Pantera and Megadeth and never missed a workout or a meal, ever. For a few weeks there was little to no change. I never wavered. After a few more weeks, pants were slightly looser. And then finally, clients began asking what I was doing and definitely noticed a difference. They motivated me, their trainer, far more than I could ever hope to motivate them.

When other people chimed in with praise or even thought I was getting too skinny or assumed I was sick, I thanked them, said I was getting lean, not skinny. I told them to watch out for November 3, 2013, when they would see something in me they had not seen before. And the closer the date came, the more intensely I trained, the more focused I became. I'd engaged in a private war, and no matter what, I would win.

One day in particular when on the phone with my mother, I snarled, "If this is the last thing I accomplish, I will be in shape for this project." She immediately voiced concern about it possibly being the last thing I would ever do. I explained that sometimes things take on such a level of importance that the thought of failure is eradicated from the mind. I told her that's where my mind needed to be in order to achieve what I set out to do. I could feel her nodding over the phone—and then she suggested I go eat something.

YOU HAVE CONTROL

I want to remind you that your body is one of the few things in life that you have control over. It doesn't matter what your current weight or composition is. It doesn't matter what others are saying. It doesn't even matter what you have settled for or accepted as your best deep within the recesses of your mind. You are going to do this. You have the power to do this. You are doing this for yourself and for no one else. You will get back on that horse and get to the finish line any way you can.

Motivation must remain as continuous as blood to the heart, or the pulse will deaden. Whatever it takes for you to stay on target, you owe it to yourself to do. On one particular night during the preparation of this book, I was almost critically hungry and desiring a cheat meal so wildly that Domino's and its competition almost got the double order. Yet a simple posting on a social media site generated an influx of supportive cheers from believers and fellow journeymen, which satiated my hunger better than any pizza could.

Peering into the future has been an immense help to me. Although an immediate cheat meal would invoke feelings of temporary ecstasy, the aftermath wouldn't look pretty. I saw bloating and an upset stomach for the following day, worsened by the emotional turmoil disappointing myself would stir up. It would be too high a price to pay for immediate weakness. My philosophy is to never wake up and wonder where the day will take you. Take it to your planned destination.

Stay strong!

ON CRAVINGS

Cravings can be very frustrating to deal with while peaking your body. Since the equation of minimal fat coupled with lean body mass is the ideal but not the norm, they are your body's way of saying, "Feed me!" In the end, cravings are just like getting a shot—they're inevitable, so learn to face up to them.

Here are five things you can do to lessen the mental anguish of cravings:

- Make sure that you are getting in enough quality calories and good fats during the day to keep yourself energized and satiated.
- Use spices to add variety to foods.
- Remember that once per week you've got your cheat meal coming up.
- Put yourself in the line of fire: Take your shirt off right now and look at your image in the mirror. Would you be confident with this same image on your social media site right now for all to see as your profile pic? For me this is usually a good indicator and powerful enough to keep me on my program.
- Give yourself crystal-clear reminders of what you are trying to achieve, your end goal, your event, your peak day.

What follows is a small list of foods that I turn to when the mental burden of staying on track can seem overwhelming. It's my staple of small pleasures, without the guilt.

- Frozen diet soda or ice pops
- Lettuce
- Pickles (avoid if you have high blood pressure)
- Egg-white omelet

ENDGAME

When I relocated to Los Angeles, one of the first things I heard was, "You don't fail, you quit." As long as we keep plugging away, we are active players in the game. And in your new world, the only place that true failure will occur (or should occur) is in the gym, when you hit the point of positive muscular failure when temporarily no further repetitions are possible. That's *good* failure. And the *only* place that you are allowed to fail.

It is not important that you assemble all the components in front of you. It is not important that everything gets done perfectly and at the same time. It is important that you do the best you can and commit to yourself. It is important to stay motivated and on track. It is important that you believe and know that only you have the power to change yourself for the better, that this is actually a tangible thing that you are in control of.

Remember what brought you to the conclusion that your current self didn't represent your best self and how you truly wish to see yourself and what drove you to take action in the first place. Treat not your body like that of a new book or DVD that had to be purchased and yet was never read or watched. To this goal you shall meet. The desire, belief, call to action and will is the only thread that you will ever need to cross the river of victory. Turn excuse and problematic into endurable and promising.

Burst through the finish line with more intensity than when you began. Now, get back on your horse and ride!

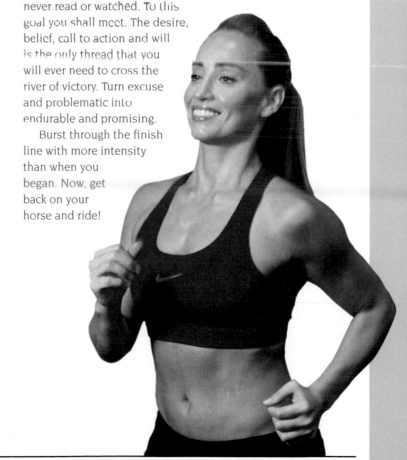

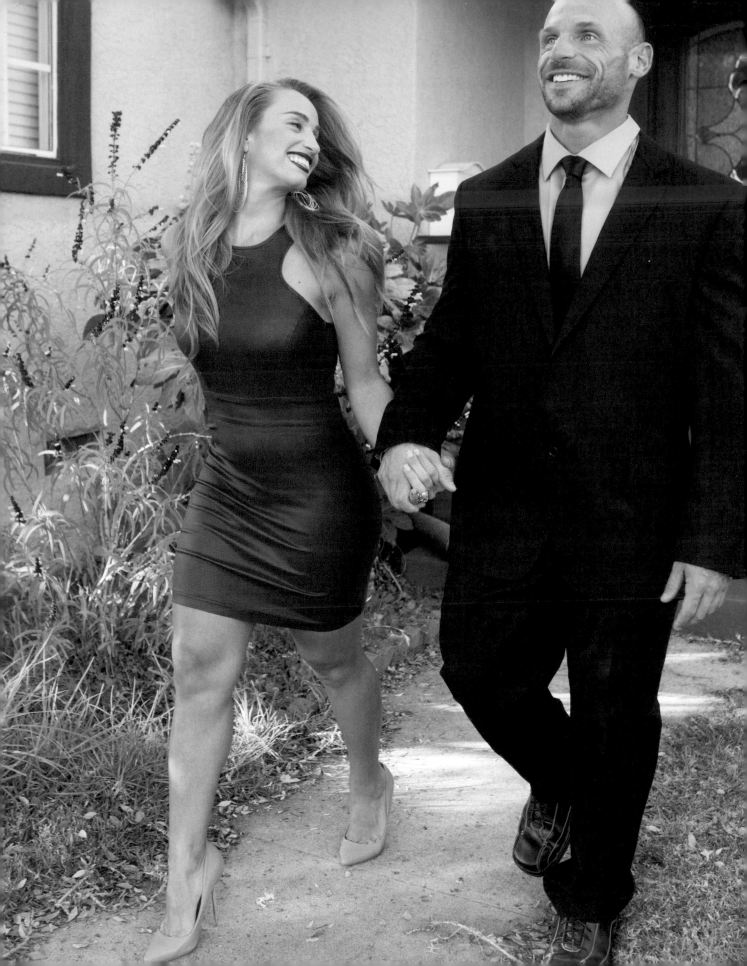

CHAPTER 9

'HELLO MY NAME IS' . . . AND BEYOND

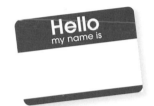

If you've made it this far, then you've made it to the big dance, and I want to congratulate you.

For, since you first began your Peak Physique program, you have become truly better in not only physique on the outside but also better inside as a human being.

And now that your motivation, desire and need have carried you to this long-awaited day, when you can now fit into the dress or suit that you envisioned for so long, I want you to remain motivated and able to consistently fit in the dress or suit if and when the need arises. You want to stay ready for anything.

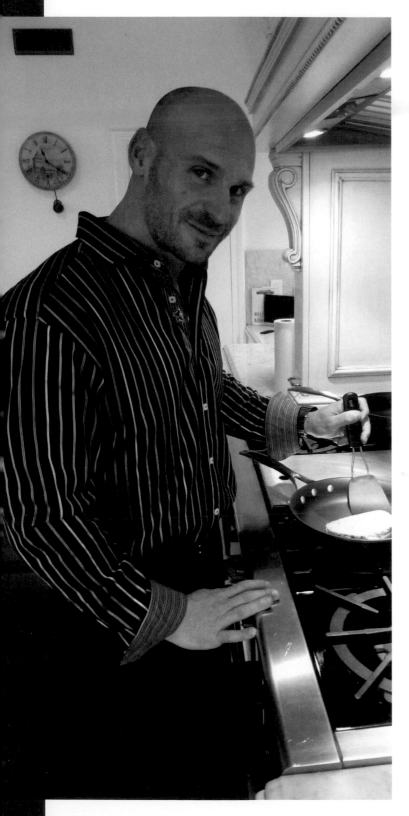

CELEBRATE!

Of course you should celebrate. Of course you should enjoy. Of course you can loosen the belt temporarily. In the movie *Carlito's Way*, Al Pacino tells us, "You can't sprint all the way. You gotta stop sometime." One can't floor the gas pedal all the time, but I do urge you to keep the engine warm and on idle.

AVOID THE YO-YO SYNDROME

All too often when attaining our physique goals, not necessarily our weight goals but body composition goals, the endless cycle of weight gain and loss catches us in an endless yo-yo syndrome. I hope I've shown you the how's and why's of getting into your best shape and also in keeping in shape following your event.

To truly succeed in any endeavor, the process must become a lifestyle, something you practice week in and week out year-round. For me, making healthy and palatable meal choices and working out are as normal and a part of my life as brushing my teeth, putting gas in the car or taking my dogs for a walk.

It is important to routinely check in with yourself. Put that dress or suit on. How is it fitting? If the holiday season is here or approaching, are you picking your spots and partaking or stashing away time while gorging and vowing to start anew at some undefined point in time? Do you keep a circle of loved ones or friends in your life who not only approve and understand your healthy lifestyle, but also implement their own form of exercise and good nutrition into their own lives? Perhaps you're already looking to the next event when the best you will be put on display, and you're not only looking to duplicate your current results, but surpass them as well.

FUTURE MAINTENANCE

So the last remaining question is this: How do you maintain this new body of yours? You hold the template in your hands, the experience in your pores and the need in your being. The next chapter has yet to be written, but it starts with you.

In closing, I leave you with two important thoughts: That looking beyond the instant gratification of the world in which we live in today will help to keep you grounded in the concrete steps of tomorrow, and that we have very little direct control in our lives but our body and its physical workings are well within our grasp to make the most of and run efficiently over a lifetime. Thank you for picking up the journey with me. I'll see you where real results happen: in the gym and at the dinner table.

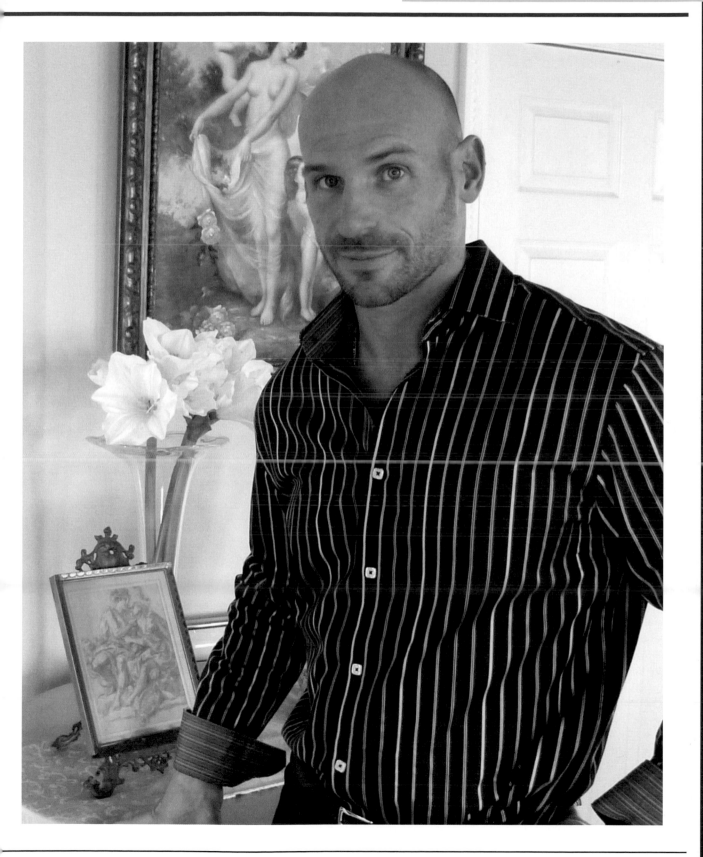

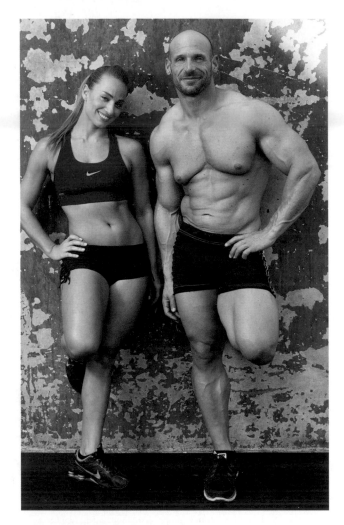

Before his career as author and personal trainer, HOLLIS LANCE LIEBMAN has been a fitness magazine editor, national bodybuilding champion and published physique photographer, and he has also served as a bodybuilding and fitness competition judge. Currently a Los Angeles resident, Hollis has worked with some of Hollywood's elite, earning himself rave reviews. *Peak Physique* is his eighth book.

Visit www.holliswashere.com for fitness tips and complete training programs.

Twitter: @hllpac

Facebook: holliswashere.com

Instagram: HLLPAC

YouTube: Hollis Liebman

CREDITS

Editorial and design by Lisa Purcell Editorial & Design (purcelleditorial.com)

Photography by Jen Schmidt (jenschmidtphotography.com)

Female model: Michelle Brooke (www.blocagency.com/)

Majority of men's clothing provided by (www.gorillawearonline.com)

Photographed on location at Gold's Gym, Venice, California, USA (www.goldsgym.com/veniceca/)

Recipes and food images supplied by The Life Chef (www.lalifechef.com)

All photos by Jen Schmidt, except the following: *page 9 (inset)* iqoncept/CanStockPhoto; 16 leremy/CanStockPhoto; 23 izaphoto/CanStockPhoto; 24 dencg/CanStockPhoto; 29 sbotas/CanStockPhoto; 35 *middle* Sun Ladder/Wikimedia Commons; 35 *bottom* Mullookkaaran/Wikimedia Commons; 35 *right* Evan-Amos/Wikimedia Commons; 36 *top left* Raeky/Wikimedia Commons; 36 *bottom left* draghicich/CanStockPhoto; 36 *top right* Alex011973/CanStockPhoto; 36 *bottom right* noblige/CanStockPhoto; 37 *left* baibaz/CanStockPhoto; 45 Jef Poskanzer/Wikimedia Commons

ABOUT THE MODEL

Michelle Brooke, a native of Brooklyn, New York, is a passionate creative director, choreographer, performer and world-wide instructor of dance and dance fitness. Her accomplishments throughout her career include working with most of today's top artists and TV shows and creating Dance Exposed Productions, which offers unique and innovative creativity in all forms of dance and entertainment for productions, tours, TV shows, films, commercials, music videos, industrials, PVT events and Domestic/International Workshops & Master classes (www.DanceeXposed.com). You can visit her website at www.MichelleBrooke.com

Twitter: @Michelle_Brooke

Instagram: michellebrookelyn Bodfitness

ACKNOWLEDGEMENTS

The author wishes to thank the good people of Gold's Gym, Venice, CA; Gorilla Wear; and especially the tireless efforts of Lisa Purcell and Jen Schmidt.

Somewhere right now a young boy or girl is thumbing through their first fitness magazine and, without knowing it, has just been bitten by the iron bug. It is to you, the next generation of iron warrior, who this book is dedicated to, for you will carry and then one day pass the torch. Share what you have learned.